Human Fertility in Latin America
Sociological Perspectives

HUMAN FERTILITY
IN LATIN AMERICA

Sociological Perspectives

J. MAYONE STYCOS

Cornell University Press

ITHACA, NEW YORK

Copyright © 1968 by Cornell University

First published 1968

Library of Congress Catalog Card Number: 68-14115

PRINTED IN THE UNITED STATES OF AMERICA
BY VAIL-BALLOU PRESS, INC.

MARYSI I NASZEMU DZIECKU

Foreword

by Dudley Kirk

Nowhere in the world has the population "explosion" occurred with greater force than in Latin America. In population (though not in economic development) Latin America is the most rapidly growing major region in the world.

This rapid population growth is well documented in national censuses, and it is recognized that the rapid growth is caused by a widespread and desirable reduction in the death rate, without parallel reduction in the high birth rate of the region. But why is fertility in Latin America so high? What forces are working for lower birth rates, what against? The answers are often glib, speculative, and more in the realm of folklore than of fact.

Professor Stycos has devoted much of his professional life to the objective study of these questions. He has lived and worked in both Puerto Rico and Jamaica, and in both countries he has participated in major field studies on the knowledge, attitudes, and practices relating to family size and family limitation. These studies were among the first to show the feasibility of getting valid information on such delicate subjects in underdeveloped areas through household interviews. His publication (with Kurt W. Back) on the pitfalls and methodology of such interviewing has been of great value to later inquiries in many other countries.

From his early work in Puerto Rico, he developed the theory of "machismo" as an explanation of high fertility. His later research led him to retract this hypothesis, despite the wide popularity it received, in favor of the more sophisticated sociological explanations presented in this book.

Professor Stycos has supervised attitude studies on fertility and fertility control in Peru, Colombia, and Haiti; he had an important role in planning the series of studies, coordinated by the United Nations Latin American Demographic Centre, of factors affecting fertility in eight Latin American cities.

While Professor Stycos is author, co-author, and editor of several books dealing with Latin American population studies, much of his work has been published in widely scattered sources. And several of the eighteen papers here brought together in orderly sequence have not previously been published at all.

In these papers Professor Stycos brings the findings of his empirical studies to bear on many problems not immediately evident from the chapter titles. Why is the Latin American intellectual less aware of and less concerned about population problems than his counterpart elsewhere? Why has the medical profession taken the lead in promoting family planning in Latin America (in sharp contrast with the United States and Europe)? What is the role of the Church—is fertility high because of its dicta, or is its influence more on verbalized attitudes than on actual fertility? What is the influence of political ideologies, both left and right, on attitudes toward birth control? To what extent are Latin American attitudes on fertility control influenced (positively and negatively) by the activities of North Americans and of the U.S. Government? Why is the influence of voluntary organizations so weak? What are the channels of influence and communication that might bring change?

In his discussion of these topics Professor Stycos is always prepared to confront and present the basic issues in direct language. As a sociologist, he also evaluates the influence on fertility of Latin American social norms and structure. What is the effect of unstable family relationships on fertility? Is promiscuity a cause of high fertility? Does the employment of women reduce their fertility? Is it true that education and urbanization have less influence in reducing fertility in Latin America than in other parts of the world? And what, finally, are the prospects for fertility control in Latin America?

Professor Stycos discusses these issues with the warmth of one who knows Latin America well—its culture, its language, indeed its music, in which he is an able performer. In this book readers will find the quantitative results of scientific inquiry combined with the perceptive insights of an experienced and sympathetic observer.

The book is intended for Latin American as well as North American readers; Spanish and Portuguese editions are in preparation.

New York City
May 1967

Acknowledgments

In a collection of papers spanning more than a decade, it is only fitting that I pay at least some of the interest on my intellectual debts. Kingsley Davis early sparked my motivation to study human fertility, both by intellectual stimulation at Princeton and Columbia, and by hiring me as highly unskilled labor on a survey of Puerto Rican fertility in 1947. The cultural shock at this first exposure to Latin American society can best be described as ecstasy. Subsequently, Paul Lazarsfeld, Dean Manheimer, and others at Columbia University's Bureau of Applied Social Research caused me to appreciate how flexible a research tool the social survey can be. Thus armed with both Mission and Method, I repeatedly set sail for various parts of the New World.

Like earlier voyagers to these uncharted territories, I found that a great deal of the expeditions' energies must be devoted to the location of suitable patrons. In this connection I am most grateful for the courageous sponsorship of the Conservation Foundation and the Population Council, in the days when research on family planning was viewed as risky, if not risqué.

Portions of the book have appeared elsewhere, and I would like to thank the following journals and publishers for permission to reprint: in Chapter 1, from "The Outlook for World Population," *Science*, CXLVI (December 11, 1964), copyright 1964 by the American Association for the Advancement of

ACKNOWLEDGMENTS

Science; and from "Birth Control: The Restrictions of the Western Approach," *Lancet* (December 11, 1965); in Chapter 2, from "Population Problems in Latin America: A Hemisphere Perspective," *Journal of Family Welfare* (India), XI, No. 2 (December 1964); in Chapter 3, from "Opinion of Latin American Intellectuals on Population Problems and Birth Control," *Annals of the American Academy of Political and Social Sciences*, CCCLX (July 1965); in Chapters 3 and 18, from "Demography and the Study of Population Problems in Latin America," *Population Dilemma in Latin America*, edited by J. M. Stycos and J. Arias (Colombia Books, 1966); in Chapter 4, from "Survey Research and Population Control in Latin America," *Public Opinion Quarterly*, XXVIII (Fall 1964); in Chapter 5, from "Birth Control Clinics in Crowded Puerto Rico," *Health, Culture, and Community*, edited by B. Paul (Russell Sage Foundation, 1955); in Chapter 6, from "Interpersonal Influence in Family Planning in Puerto Rico" (with K. W. Back and R. Hill), *Transactions of the Third World Conference of Sociology* (International Sociological Association), VIII (1956); in Chapter 8, from "Attitudes toward Family Size in Haiti," *Human Organization* (Society for Applied Sociology), XXIII (Spring 1964); in Chapter 9, from "Experiments in Social Change: The Caribbean Fertility Studies," *Research in Family Planning*, edited by C. V. Kiser (Princeton University Press, 1962); in Chapter 10, from "Family Size Preferences and Social Class in Peru," *American Journal of Sociology*, LXX (May 1965); in Chapter 11, from "Contraception and Catholicism in Latin America," *Journal of Social Issues* (Fall 1967); in Chapter 12, from J. M. Stycos and K. W. Back, *The Control of Human Fertility in Jamaica* (Cornell University Press, 1964); in Chapter 14, from "Culture and Differential Fertility in Peru," *Population Studies*, XVI (March 1963); and in Chapters 15 and 17, from "Female Employment and Fertility in Lima, Peru," *Milbank Memorial Fund Quarterly*, XLIII, No. 1 (January 1965), and "Needed Research in Latin American Fertility: Urbanization and Fertility," *ibid.*, No. 4, Pt. 2 (October 1965).

J. MAYONE STYCOS

Cornell University
August 1967

Contents

*¿Dónde están las fronteras entre espasmo y terremoto,
entre erupción y cohabitación?*

Octavio Paz

I

A GENERAL VIEW

1

Population Control
in World Perspective

There are at least two remarkable and unprecedented aspects to the population problem today—the first is the rate of population growth, the second is the growing inclination on the part of national governments to manipulate this rate.

Rapid population growth was characteristic of most European countries in the past century, and much of the excess population found its way to the New World. But rates of growth in underdeveloped areas today, ranging from about 2 to 3.5 percent per year, are about twice those of European countries during the period of their most rapid growth. A population growing at the rate of 3 percent per year will double in 23 years, and one growing at the rate of 2 percent in 35 years. Since the population bases in the underdeveloped areas today far exceed those of Europe, the implications in sheer numbers of a rapid rate of growth are truly impressive. For example, if India alone were to grow for the next century somewhat more slowly than it is growing now, it would still have millions more inhabitants than the entire world has today.

The basic ingredients of this growth are by now well known. Low death rates, which it took European countries a century to a century and a half to achieve, are being approached in underdeveloped areas in a fifth of the time, but birth rates, which it took Europe sixty to seventy years to bring down to modern levels, show little sign of decline.

Various kinds of concern are expressed about the "population explosion." Some people seem concerned about sheer physical space and cite figures to show that there will be "standing room only" at some future date. Others see the increase as outrunning food resources or as hastening the end of our nonrenewable resources. Some are convinced that the increase spells genetic disaster, others are esthetically revolted by human crowding, and still others see it as a cause of wars. All such arguments, while they may have some truth, have serious limitations and in any event have had little impact on policy makers in underdeveloped areas. But there is one general line of reasoning which is having a major impact on leaders in the underdeveloped areas: it is demonstrable that current rates of population growth are slowing down economic development and that a reduction in the rate of growth would have substantial salutary consequences for the economy. This argument does not imply that population control is a substitute for the usual ingredients of modernization—education, industrialization, technological development, and so forth —but that it will enable underdeveloped countries to take full advantage of such developments and make it possible for them to add to their per capita wealth and productivity.

It can be shown that high rates of population growth impair economic development by requiring higher proportions of national income to be saved and invested merely to maintain current levels of per capita income. Further, because of the large proportions of young people in high fertility nations, capital is diverted from productive channels to consumption and to social services. But in underdeveloped countries, even social services are having an increasingly difficult time in making per capita gains, when *new* population tends to occupy the new houses, classrooms, and hospitals.

The consequences for economic development of rapid population growth and of changes in population age structures have only recently been defined in a scientific fashion, and are only slowly coming to the attention of national governments. For most of man's history, rapid population growth has been regarded as a sign of national vitality, as a basis of military and political power, as a source of a cheap labor, and as a stimulus for internal markets. Many current national anticontraceptive laws and family allowance programs in Europe stem from post-World War I fears of population decline. To these older philosophies has been added that of the new nation desiring a place in the sun, a place assured only if there are enough people to occupy it.

The recent upsurge of interest in the relation between economic development and population growth has various causes. Despite bootstrap efforts and foreign aid, most underdeveloped countries have been unable to make substantial gains in per capita income since the war. Further, the postwar period has seen the establishment in many countries of planning boards and commissions whose task it is to assess future national needs and to plan policies accordingly. The importance of these boards cannot be overestimated for, in the broadest sense, their existence implies that rationality in human affairs is not only possible but desirable. It further implies that economic and social variables should be manipulated to meet future needs in the service of modernization and that a professional group can legitimately advise on or implement such manipulation. Where such groups are conscientious they cannot avoid looking at population growth estimates, since the number of jobs, schools, hospitals, roads, and so forth needed in the next five or ten years is partly fixed by the population size expected at that time. On looking, the planners sometimes cannot believe their eyes and call for foreign experts, an improvement in their statistical and census services, or both. But the second look is often worse than the first, since inadequate statistical facilities tend to give too low, rather than too high, an estimate of growth rates. Disbelief then often turns to alarm. A solution which is perhaps not so unique was cited at a recent international conference, where the deputy head of Pakistan's Planning Commission admitted ruefully that the 1.4 percent growth rate assumed for their 1955–1960 five-year plan had been calculated "to keep despair away. We are all convinced that population is growing faster than that."

Some countries, including Pakistan, do more than despair, and take steps to slow down the rate of population growth. There are only three ways in which this can be done—by raising the death rate, lowering the birth rate, or increasing the rate of migration. Since it is neither humane nor politic to slow down the decline in the death rate, this solution is rarely discussed, although eventually some countries may be pushed into considering it. International migration is almost as unfeasible a solution. Since most countries today are worried about their own population growth, few are interested in adding to it with foreigners. In any event, population growth today is of such dimensions that migration as a solution is impracticable. Every year, for example, there are ten million more Indians than in the previous year. What then of birth rates?

SHORT-RUN PROSPECTS OF FERTILITY DECLINE

Many leaders in underdeveloped areas believe that economic development and urbanization will bring down birth rates "as they did in Europe without explicit policies." Leaving aside the obvious point that the population growth is slowing down the very economic growth which is supposed to check it, it is probable that in some unspecified "long run" birth rates will in fact decline. (Of course, in a period when the peoples of underdeveloped areas are in a hurry for the goods and skills of the modern world, to leave any solution to the "long run" is both politically inexpedient and ethically questionable.) But in the short run there are reasons for believing that "letting nature take its course" may leave fertility much where it is today. Historically, birth rates responded only slowly to the processes of modernization. In the late nineteenth century, European populations were characterized by higher literacy and less rigid social stratification than are typical for most underdeveloped areas today. People married at relatively late ages, and the birth rates were considerably below those of the underdeveloped areas today. Despite these favorable conditions, it took European countries 60 to 70 years to bring their birth rates down to modern levels. The dimensions of today's problem are considerable. Births in underdeveloped areas average 40 to 45 per year for every 1,000 population. To bring this rate down to the 17 to 20 per 1,000 characteristic of Europe would mean an annual reduction of fifty million births.

There is no magic about the relation between economic development and fertility decline. It operated in certain ways in the West and cannot be assumed to be automatic. Probably the greatest part of the decline in most countries can be attributed to deliberate efforts by couples to restrict their number of children because of the decreasing advantages and increasing disadvantages of having large families. But the use of birth control is not the only factor which affects the birth rate. The birth rate of a society is determined by other factors, such as the nutritional level, the proportions single, widowed, and divorced, the age at marriage, the frequency of sexual intercourse, the incidence of individual sterility and infertility, and the extent of lactation. While the birth rate of underdeveloped areas is high relative to that of Western nations, it by no means approaches the biological limit. Under ideal conditions the average woman can have about twelve live births; but in most underdeveloped areas the average does not exceed seven. India is a good example. By the end of childbearing, the average woman has had between six and seven live births, and the average period between the birth of one child and another is about three years. The incidence of birth control practice is so low that it cannot possibly account for this, but there are a number of aspects to Indian culture which might. Among these are the custom of the wife returning to her parents' village for an extended period after the birth of a child; the custom of breast feeding children; customs which forbid sexual relations on various ceremonial days and for a period after the birth of a child; and the low nutritional level.

The most significant point here is that all the above conditions can be expected to decline or disappear with economic development.

In other regions there are other relevant patterns. In the Caribbean the instability of marital unions has had a marked negative effect on fertility, and in other areas taboos on the remarriage of widows have had a similar effect. In most countries the number of people who live through their entire reproductive period is increasing. Indeed, recent historical investigations indicate the probability that in most European countries fertility rose in the last century before it declined. Although the data are somewhat deficient, it is perhaps significant that in the last decade a number of countries, especially in the Western Hemisphere, have shown increases in birth rates, while very few have shown declines. This has been a period when most countries have made at least modest advances in economic and social development. Thus, the short run holds little hope for "natural" decreases in birth rates as a result of economic development. Is there any chance that declines can be induced?

One of the principal reasons for optimism here is that, for the first time in history, national governments and major national institutions are devoting substantial resources to this problem. It must be remembered that the decline in birth rates in Europe and England occurred *despite* the concerted opposition of church and state, and that the culture of the nineteenth century militated against the spread of information and ideas on family planning. In many underdeveloped nations, non-Christian religions forbid neither birth control nor its discussion, and the vast prestige and resources of the state may be marshalled to spread the practice of birth control. Thus, the governments of India, Pakistan, Honduras and Korea sponsor active programs; Malaysia, Ceylon, Hong Kong, Barbados, Puerto Rico, and Chile have programs sanctioned by the government; and Taiwan, Tunisia, Turkey, the United Arab Republic, and Colombia have pilot programs in progress as preliminaries to the formation of national policies.

BIRTH CONTROL AND DEATH CONTROL

While it is a major step for governments to introduce national programs of family planning, it by no means guarantees that the problem has been solved. So far it has proved far more difficult to reduce fertility than to reduce mortality. There are several reasons for this.

(1) Technology in family planning has been primitive compared to medical technology as a whole. This is largely the result of the poor state of scientific knowledge concerning reproductive physiology, a situation which presents an interesting question for the sociology of science.

(2) The most effective public health procedures are directed at communities rather than individuals and thus avoid the problems of individual decision-making. Highly successful public health methods, such as mass DDT spraying, sewage control, and water filtration, have no parallels in fertility control, where individual couples must normally make frequent and continual decisions to apply contraceptive technology.

(3) Mortality control methods are in the service of goals which are universally shared—the prolongation of life, the alleviation of pain, the prevention and care of disease. Fertility control may be running counter to deep-seated motivations. Children provide prestige, amusement, religious blessing, social security, and pleasure in most societies, and, where infant mortality is high, the society must encourage high fertility in order to guarantee perpetuation.

While these considerations render fertility control a more difficult problem than mortality control, a number of recent advances in knowledge have provided grounds for optimism. For

9

example, over the past decade there has been a certain amount of favorable evidence concerning the efficacy and acceptability of unconventional methods of fertility control—sterilization, abortion, and intrauterine devices.

UNCONVENTIONAL METHODS

Surveys of public opinion in underdeveloped areas indicate that women develop a strong interest in birth control only after they have had several children. They have little interest in spacing children, but once they have their desired number they wish to stop having children. Sterilization is the ideal technique for such individuals. It has the additional advantages of being easy to talk about, since, unlike most contraceptives, it does not require references to the sexual act or sexual organs. Finally, it is performed in a hospital, thus partaking of the aura of prestige and safety to health which contraceptives lack for many. Since it is normally a postpartum operation requiring only a few additional days in the hospital after delivery, it can be accomplished inconspicuously. The widespread use of this method in such differing cultures as Puerto Rico and India show that what appears to be a drastic solution to many middle class people can be a swift and simple solution to lower-income groups.

Sterilization of males is an even more promising technique, for it is a simpler operation which does not require hospitalization. Certain of the states of India are promoting this approach, utilizing mobile camp techniques and offering the men small subsidies (10 to 30 rupees) and transportation facilities. The demand for this technique has exceeded the expectation of most Indian experts—between 1956 and 1963 at least 240,000 male operations were performed. Whereas in 1957 there were about three female for every male sterilization, in 1962 there were three male for every female sterilization.

Abortion is another technique which Americans tend to regard as drastic, unethical, or dangerous to health; but in other countries it is considered none of these and is highly popular as well. With the exception of East Germany and Albania, all the Communist countries in Europe have official abortion programs. In Czechoslovakia and Hungary for example, there were 7 and 17 abortions respectively for every 1,000 population in 1961. In the latter country there were more officially recorded abortions than births. In all the countries which have such programs, birth rates have declined markedly in recent years.

Abortion has the advantage of being required only when a pregnancy is absolutely certain. It requires no foresight, planning, or interference with the sexual act. Under proper medical supervision the risk is little greater than the risk of a tonsilectomy. Both medically supervised abortion and sterilization, then, avoid to a considerable degree the problems associated with repeated decision-making around the time of the sexual act. On the other hand, since they require skilled personnel, they are relatively expensive; most sterilizations are irreversible and cannot be used for child spacing; and repeated abortions are a greater health hazard than are standard contraceptives.

Virtually all the advantages of these methods and none of their disadvantages are present with certain contraceptive methods currently under test. The most promising are the intrauterine devices. Easily produced for a few cents each, these plastic devices once inserted may need to be removed only when the woman wishes to become pregnant. Current tests indicate they may be left alone for at least two years, have a high rate of effectiveness, and cause problems with only a small minority of women. While they must be inserted under aseptic conditions by trained persons, this can probably be done by paramedical personnel such as midwives and nurses. Thus, the intrauterine devices are a kind of cheap, easily reversible, and nonoperative sterilization.

THE DESIRED FAMILY SIZE

While there is doubtless a crude inverse correlation between the simplicity of the method and the degree of motivation required for its adoption, even the simplest method requires some interest. It has been claimed repeatedly that the general population in underdeveloped areas desires large families or as many children as possible or that they are totally indifferent to the number of children they have. Under such conditions any contraceptive other than a surreptitious or obligatory one (such as one put in the water by the state) is unlikely to be acceptable to enough people to have any impact on the birth rate.

Fortunately the last decade has witnessed the assembly of an extraordinary series of sample surveys which allows us to begin to answer this question. These surveys have asked more detailed and more intimate questions than are possible in the official censuses, eliciting data ranging from complete pregnancy histories to attitudes toward family size and contraception. Such studies have already been completed in 13 countries of the Western Hemisphere, 3 African, 3 Middle Eastern, 5 European, and 7 Oriental nations. According to W. Parker Mauldin, Demographic Director of the Population Council, "This is the most substantial set of comparative social data ever collected across such a range of societies, and a few of the pilot projects in the field of family planning are among the most elaborate and extensive social experiments ever carried on in the natural setting."

With respect to questions on desired number of children, the countries fall into three rough categories—those in which the average respondent wants a very large family or is indifferent to the number she has, those in which a limited but moderately large number of children are desired, and those in which a small number of children are desired.

Thus far, only a few studies have yielded responses of the first type, and they have been limited to highly underdeveloped areas —rural Africa south of the Sahara and rural Haiti.

The ideal in most countries tends to be a family of three or four children. In surveys conducted by the writer over the past decade in countries as different as Turkey, Peru, and Jamaica, most women who have two or fewer children want to have more, but most women who have three children (or more) want no more children. The reasons given by both women and men are largely economic: the high cost of clothes, food, education, and so forth, for the children.

Finally, a handful of countries, mostly European, where mortality is very low and education and income very high, express preferences for small families. In the United States about 90 percent of a national sample preferred between two and four, with the average about three and a half. Puerto Rico also falls in this category. As early as 1948, more than half of the women thought two or fewer children ideal.

NATIONAL BIRTH CONTROL PROGRAMS

While the evidence indicates an interest in having fewer children than women in fact have in most countries, it is a long and tortuous path between such verbally expressed ideals and behavior which would bring them about. While most of the studies show that the average woman has an interest in family planning, they also reveal ignorance of the most elementary facts of reproductive biology and birth control. Thus, the expressed attitudes are based on little information and little thought. The attitudes are probably not very intense, and the opinions not very salient. For many countries, the provision of technology will not be enough.

Partly for this reason, national programs of family planning have thus far shown few encouraging results; but there are other reasons. The early programs of several countries tended to copy the administrative, technical, and philosophical orientation of the planned parenthood movements of the United States and England, where, for historical reasons, they have been dominated by feminist, medical, and middle-class thinking. As a result, there has been heavy reliance on the person-to-person and "confidential private interview" approach typical of relations between doctor and patient or caseworker and client. On the contrary, group and community education techniques are indicated in nonpuritanical societies where a major obstacle to use of birth control is ignorance that one's peers are as favorable to the idea as oneself. There has been excessive concentration on the clinic as the major dispenser of supplies and information, with too little attention paid to commercial and other communal nonmedical distribution systems. In Western countries clinics and clinically prescribed methods have been of minimal significance in contrast with commercial (condom), folk (coitus interruptus), and extralegal (abortion) methods. In non-Western and predominantly rural countries the clinic has the special disadvantage of being most inaccessible to large sections of the very populations which most need its services. Western birth control movements and organizations have been led by women and for women, despite the fact that methods used by males are almost entirely responsible for the major declines in fertility. In non-Western societies, where the male has greater authority in the family and community than in Europe and the United States, the typical concentration of female personnel emphasizing female contraceptives seems particularly misplaced. There has also been undue emphasis on medical staffs and medical rationalizations for family planning, when in fact most people view the problem as a social and economic one. Finally, there has been virtually no attention to less direct approaches to reducing fertility, such as raising the age at marriage and encouraging female employment, discouraging cottage industry, and providing economic and social rewards for moderate fertility. But the programs are young and the nations are learning that approaches which never had much impact in

Europe and the United States can be expected to have even less in underdeveloped areas.

CHRISTIANITY AND CAPITALISM

The West has so little imaginative technical assistance to offer at the present time because we have never tried ourselves, and we are slow to learn how because we are victims of a history of thought alien to national programs of population control. Both our religious and our ideological heritages, that is, Christianity and capitalism, stand in our way.

The implications of Christianity for the development of population control in European societies refer both to the communication of ideas and to the range of methods admissible for family planning. The Christian attitude toward sex as a necessary evil has hampered seriously the spread of information on birth control. Printed literature has been scarce, of generally poor quality, and subject to severe legal restrictions. (This is in marked contrast, for example, to the situation in Japan, where a different tradition has permitted the spread of technical information through newspapers and magazines.) Radio, cinema, and television, even more limited by puritanical taboos, have had no role in the spread of information on family planning. Perhaps too characteristically, the technically magnificent channels of communication in the West have been devoid of content. So seriously restricted is technical knowledge on contraception, that the average general practitioner in England and the United States has had little exposure to it. Many of the people of underdeveloped nations are illiterate, but few are deaf and blind. The provision of audio-visual materials holds more promise and more feasibility than the provision of physicians, nurses, or social workers. Unfortunately, however, apart from the purely technical aspects, in the area of communications the only experience the West has to offer underdeveloped countries is bad experience.

Christianity has also affected our attitude toward methods. It is paradoxical that the methods most universally known—abortion and coitus interruptus, have been the methods most vigorously condemned. Because of the Christian view of the soul, the former method is usually seen as a form of murder, and the latter, due to an unfortunate combination of biblical circumstances, as the sin of Onanism. Even the medical profession and family planners have often raised their voices to condemn these techniques, ostensibly because of their inefficiency and danger to health, but more accurately because they never seemed "normal" or "ethical," according to middle-class Western standards.

Finally, there has been an influential notion that by removing the threat of pregnancy, contraceptives are increasing promiscuity. While there is little evidence one way or the other on this question, the idea that unwanted children are preferable to non-marital sexual relations seems particularly Christian, and is not one we should be particularly eager to make available for export.

The Western system of private enterprise has had a number of interesting consequences for population control, especially in connection with voluntary organizations and the profession of medicine.

Under the general philosophy of "that government is best which governs least," the capitalist society leaves to private enterprise a great many activities in health and social welfare which are assumed by the state in other forms of government. Thus the phenomenon, unfathomable to the foreigner, of a multitude of American private organizations, devoted to solving, by means of voluntary contributions of time and money, problems such as polio, cerebral palsy, heart disease, tuberculosis, mental disorder, alcoholism, traffic accidents, cruelty to animals, and birth control. In the United States voluntary agencies often operate alongside of functionally similar government agencies, and are almost invariably well financed, due to the American belief in large charitable contributions and small taxes. Thus it comes as no surprise that such an important sphere of health and welfare as family planning has private and voluntary agencies devoted to its promotion. The surprises are rather that there are no parallel government agencies devoted to the problem, and that the volunteer agencies for family planning are both poorly financed and poorly staffed.

Because of the Christian ideological opposition to sex discussion in general and family planning in particular, these organizations have not only had difficulty in extracting contributions from Americans already deluged with requests for assistance on noncontroversial problems, but have attracted highly atypical segments of society as leaders and members. Both in the United States and England the movements have tended to collect people long on fire and combativeness and short on organizational ability. This is a perfectly natural situation in the early days of any movement; only after it achieves power and respectability do the establishment types take over. Unfortunately, the birth control movement has never fully achieved power or respectability in England or the United States, and perhaps for this reason has never had much impact in terms of services. In Great Britain, for example, less than one of every ten users of birth control has ever received advice from a family planning clinic, and the chances are that the patient paid for such advice. So modest are their services that half the net income of British family planning clinics is derived from the sale of contraceptives.

Given their history and present circumstances then, does England or the United States have anything to teach India or Latin America? All we have to demonstrate are our relatively low birth rates, and for all we usefully know about them they might have been produced by magic. Indeed, achieved as they were in the face of such odds, they *are* little short of miraculous, and reflect the responsibility and persistence of individual couples, rather than of governments, voluntary organizations, or physicians.

There are several limitations of traditional Western medicine as applied to underdeveloped areas. First, Western medicine has always been more attracted by the pound of cure than by the ounce of prevention. Second, there has been an emphasis on maximum attention and treatment for the individual private patient rather than on mass approaches. Thus clinical medicine usually has more prestige than public health, and a certain mystique about the necessity for a close doctor-patient relation emerges. The average physician knows surprisingly little about contraception, and the little he knows he tends to guard closely. There is among many of the profession a feeling that public service or educational programs on birth control are somehow inappropriate. Knowledge of such matters is the property of the doctor, who must dispense it with discrimination by means of face-to-face relations in the sanctity of his office. Moreover, excluding birth control from the normal services of hospitals and other health facilities gives family planning an aura of distinctiveness it can ill afford. Whatever their benefits in rich nations, such approaches are not only economically unfeasible in poor nations, but especially inefficacious. There is, in short, an *ambiance* about medicine and birth control in most rich nations which it were better the student from the underdeveloped country did not absorb.

Newly emerging countries do not have to produce steam engines before they produce jets, and there is no reason why they cannot avoid the ignoble and bitter experience of the wealthy nations with respect to birth control. Most of the newer nations do not have a Christian tradition to deal with, and in the only major exception, Latin America, the twentieth-century Catholic Church bears little resemblance to the nineteenth-century Church with regard to family planning. Nor is there the danger that the emergence of volunteer organizations will allow governments to evade their responsibilities, since volunteer organizations are especially weak. Moreover, since there is a firm belief in the active role of the government in the process of modernization, there is little danger that solutions of health problems will be left to amateurs and crusading enthusiasts.

Indeed, with such potential advantages it may be that poorer countries need moral assistance as urgently as technical. We can give this only by putting our house in order—by recognizing family planning services as a normal component of the general health responsibilities of government, and mass family planning education as a normal part of the general educational responsibilities of government.

Newly developing countries have demographic aims the scope of which the West has never seen nor dreamed of. Pakistan's newest five-year plan calls for a 20 percent reduction of the birth rate by means of ten million insertions of intrauterine devices at a cost of two dollars per insertion. Tunisia plans 120,000 insertions in the next two years, Korea 200,000, Turkey 500,000, and so on. These are jet-age programs unhaunted by moral and technological ghosts of earlier times. In the technical assistance area, probably the major contribution we can make at this time is training in the scientific method applied to medical, educational, and organizational aspects of family planning programs. Scientifically sound evaluation programs, in conjunction with imaginative programmatic innovations will provide the underdeveloped area with powerful tools for solution of population problems. A judicious combination of native hypotheses and technically assisted evaluation procedures should provide the necessary breakthroughs.

THE ROLE OF RESEARCH

Indeed, the need for research on the demographic, biomedical, and sociopsychological aspects of the population problem is one of the most pressing scientific demands today. Ignorance in this field is very great. For example, probably fewer than half of the world's births and a third of its deaths are registered; thus we have only crude estimates of the vital rates of most of the world, and we have least knowledge about those countries for which demographic knowledge is needed most.

In another research area, the intrauterine devices are proving to be among the cheapest, safest, simplest, and most effective contraceptives ever developed; yet so elementary is our knowledge about basic physiology of reproduction that how these devices work is unknown. (Hudson Hoagland, President of the American Academy of Arts and Sciences, states that "as a result of prudery about sex, and of religious and political opposition to birth control, investigators have not been encouraged to enter the very important field of mammalian reproduction.")

Finally, while we know a good deal in some countries about the social characteristics (religion, income, education, and so forth) of people who practice birth control as opposed to those who do not, we are virtually ignorant of the social psychological processes which impel one family to adopt family planning and another not to.

But serious attention to the population problem is new. The Population Council, the principal organization devoted to supporting research in this area, was founded only in 1952, and as late as 1960 had a total budget of only $2.7 million (although this had increased to $7.3 million by 1967). The major foundations have announced significant support for population research only within the past few years. In 1961, the National Institutes of Health, which expended $880 million on control of fatalities, expended only $1.3 million on research relating to fertility control. Only a handful of universities are producing demographers, and virtually no psychologists, anthropologists, or political scientists have turned their attention to population problems. American government agencies are only beginning to give official recognition to the problem, and international agencies such as the United Nations and the World Health Organization are circling the problem seriously, but gingerly.

In short, major attention to population dynamics is in its infancy. In the next decade we can expect breakthroughs not only of a scientific nature, but in successful national programs of population control.

2

Population Problems in Latin America: A Hemispheric Perspective

During World War I, a phrase was born which still has an impact partly based on numbers: "Forty million Frenchmen can't be wrong." The saying has a logic all its own based on the glory and power of France and its many millions of citizens (the French population was more than four times greater than that of England at the time of its industrial revolution). How does forty million sound today, in the midst of spectacular world population increase?

In the past 25 years (1940–1965) Brazil has added forty million people to its population, and in the next 15 years will add that many *more*. Latin America as a whole will add three times this number to its population in the next 15 years. Or to move the comparison from France to the Iberian Peninsula, every five years Latin America is adding the population of Spain, and every four years Brazil is adding another Portugal. So rapid is the growth that by the end of the century there will be almost nine Latin Americans living for every one who was living in 1920, and the increase alone in the 80-year period (650 million) will exceed the present combined population of India and Pakistan.

The implications of such growth rates can be seen more clearly if we consider one country as an example. The Republic of El Salvador, the smallest of the Latin American nations, is also the most densely settled. With nearly three million people living on 21,000 square kilometers, it is one of the few nations in our hemisphere which can be called "crowded," since virtually all the arable land is occupied. Despite the fact that six of every ten persons employed are in agriculture, El Salvador's production of foodstuffs has lagged behind population increase for many years, and consequently the nation must import great quantities of food every year.

As is true for most other Latin American nations, El Salvador's population problems began earlier in the century as a result of rapidly declining death rates. In 1930, the nation's annual birth rate was no higher than it is today (between 45 and 50 births per 1000 population) but its death rate (22 per thousand) was over twice the present rate. As a result, three decades ago population in El Salvador was growing by about 35,000 persons per year. The same birth rate today on a bigger population base yields twice the number of births, but because of the precipitous decline in the death rate, there are fewer yearly deaths than in 1930. The net result is that the population is now growing by almost 100,-000 per year, or close to 4 percent a year in a nation where gross national product may be growing at 3 percent. To make these figures more realistic, let us examine their implications for just one area of the modernization process—mass education.

Like other modernizing nations, El Salvador is aspiring to raise significantly the educational level of its population. With half its adult population illiterate, over 15 cents of every dollar of government expenditure goes toward education. Even so, only 58 percent of the children aged 5–14 are enrolled in primary school, and only 14 percent of those aged 15–19 are in secondary school. Now suppose the government wished only to maintain this admittedly low level of educational achievement. Because of the growth of population in these age groups, by 1980 it would have to double the number of primary school seats and more than double the number of secondary school seats. In absolute numbers this would mean an increase of almost 334,000 seats in 20 years, with no improvement in proportions being educated.

Now suppose they set higher goals for themselves so that, by

1980, 98 percent of the primary school age group and 45 percent of the secondary school age group is attending. In this case they would have to more than triple the present number of primary seats and increase secondary enrollment almost nine times. In absolute numbers total enrollment would rise from about 324,000 in 1960 to 1,300,000 in 1980.[1] It is easy to see the difficulties facing a nation desiring progress in education during a period of rapid population growth. But where the population doubles every two decades, equally serious problems are created in other spheres such as employment, housing, and health.

HEMISPHERIC GROWTH IN POPULATION

While Latin American population growth is unusually rapid, it is by no means a unique phenomenon in this hemisphere. In fact, *both* continents of the Western Hemisphere are distinct from those of the Eastern in their extraordinary and sustained rates of population growth. North America maintained an average annual rate of growth of 3 percent per year for over a century between 1750 and 1850. Comparable rates in Latin American nations began a hundred years later, and by the end of this century the overall rate of growth for Latin American countries should rival that of the North America of centuries ago. Thus far, no other continent and probably no nation outside the hemisphere has demonstrated such rates of growth for such extended periods. Indeed the industrialized countries of Europe probably never experienced sustained population growth in excess of 1.5 percent per year.

The Western Hemisphere is also notable for its spectacular birth rates. Quebec, in Canada, in the mid-nineteenth century, had a birth rate in excess of 50 and women of completed fertility

[1] Jorge Arévalo, "Population Growth and Education," in J. M. Stycos and J. Arias, *Population Dilemma in Latin America* (Washington, D.C.: Potomac Books, 1966).

had eight to ten children on the average. The United States in the early nineteenth century had a birth rate of about 55 and the average woman had seven or eight children. While no Latin American country shows rates in excess of these, several Central American countries today have rates approximating them. Birth rates of this magnitude exceed most of those found in Asiatic or African nations, and are well above rates for England and Western European nations prior to their industrialization.

Finally, in contrast with many European and Asiatic countries, the average North or South American country is not densely populated, and the average absolute size of population of most of the countries is relatively small.

In brief, the Latin American overall demographic position, while unusual in comparison with Asia, Africa, and Europe, has much in common with the North America of an earlier period. The rapid rates of population growth, the high rates of birth, and the generally low population density all have their counter-parts in the North America of a century or more ago. However, such growth similarities should not lead us to overlook a number of crucial differences.

DENSITY AND POPULATION SIZE

Low population density figures are often cited as evidence that Latin America has no population problems. Further, the existence of large uninhabited land masses is used as evidence of the need for *larger* population. But the crucial scarcities are less in terms of space or material resources than in terms of capital, skills, and social organization. North America two centuries ago was in many ways in a more advantageous position with respect to these resources than are large parts of Latin America today. The relative flexibility of the class structure, the more even distribution of wealth, the favorable market situation, all created in North America less "social density" than in Latin America.

Those who point to wide open spaces as evidence for the need for more population might ask themselves the question: Why are there so few people there now? It is hardly the case that Latin Americans do not like to move, or are irrational about economically advantageous settlement. Since World War II migration from rural areas to the crowded cities has been phenomenal. The flight is *away* from the wide open spaces. And with good reason. Migration to the city represents an easier and more pleasant readjustment than migration to a new rural area, and is a better risk for social and economic improvement. To get people to move to rural areas requires patience, skill, and capital.

The only point in settling new areas, however, is to *increase* agricultural productivity, not to expand the numbers in unproductive agriculture. This can be done by reducing the amount of marginal land under cultivation at the same time as more productive lands are settled. But *more* population is not needed for this purpose. There are already too many people on unproductive lands, and agricultural underemployment is a serious problem in many countries. In this sense of economic productivity, agricultural land is already overpopulated. Large numbers could be removed from the land without reducing productivity. The situation can be remedied either by adding capital, skills, and improved organization to existing lands, or by removing excess rural population to more productive lands. In neither case are more people needed, but the fact is that there are more rural people all the time. Despite massive migration to urban areas, the numbers living in rural areas increase with each census. While the proportion in agriculture is decreasing in a number of countries, the actual *numbers* are not. If population growth could be slowed at the same time as more productive areas are settled, economic development would clearly be accelerated.

Quite apart from the question of density is the question of absolute number. Small countries sometimes feel the need to become great—and a large population is seen as an important aspect of greatness. It is true that population size is an ingredient of national power: large armies and large-scale industries are possible only in countries with large populations. But a large population does not guarantee these—India has neither a powerful army nor powerful industries, although it has the necessary population base for both. Indeed, it is probably fair to say that India's large population, but especially its rate of population growth, is a deterrent to its power.

Latin American countries can improve their power position in the world by regional integration plans far quicker and more economically than by expanding their own population. A common market, a regional university system, or a continental defense system will improve both national power and individual well-being far more than rapid population increase.

RATES OF POPULATION GROWTH

It is, in fact, the rate of growth rather than population size or density which is the key to the "population problem." A nation growing at 2.5 percent per year must invest 5 to 12 percent of the national income per year to maintain a constant average amount of equipment per worker. Thus a high proportion of foreign loans or domestic savings must be expended just to maintain the economic *status quo*. Improvement becomes a matter very difficult for capital scarce nations.

It is sometimes said that more people represent more consumers and therefore are a stimulus to industry. This may be true in prosperous economies but not where average income is so low that it barely covers subsistence. Five million more Peruvians in the sierra tomorrow could not add materially to the effective demand for consumer goods in Peru, and would immensely complicate Peru's economic development.

Although North America's peak rates of population increase have exceeded those of South America, they occurred at a time when the size of the population was relatively small. When North American population tripled between 1850 and 1900, it was a tripling of a mere 26 million, but when Latin American population triples between 1950 and 2000 we are referring to a population of about 200 million increasing to about 600 million. In other words, a 3 percent growth rate today has far more serious implications for population growth than it did a century ago.

A second difference in growth rates is that while a major part of North America's growth was achieved by immigration, virtually all of Latin America's is occurring by means of natural increase. Thus, while the population of the United States increased by 53 million in the latter half of the nineteenth century, at least 20 million of the 53 million added persons were immigrants from Europe. By way of contrast, when, by year 2000, Latin America has added 400 million to its 1950 population, it will virtually all be the result of the excess of birth over death.

The immigrants were in the young, economically productive age groups. Thus, the United States added millions of productive workers to its labor force without the huge cost of educating, feeding, and caring for them during their childhood and youth. Latin America, on the other hand, is grappling with huge dependent populations. The proportion of the population under 15 years of age is close to 40 percent in most Latin countries, and the relatively fewer aged do not compensate for the large numbers of younger dependents. For example, North America has about 65 persons under 15 and over 59 for every 100 persons aged 15–59, whereas in Central America and tropical South America the corresponding figure is 85.

BIRTH RATES

Migration in part also accounts for North America's early high birth rates, since the immigrants tended to be both young and from European countries and economic classes of traditionally high fertility. In Latin America, the high birth rates are indigenous; indeed, the lowest birth rates are found in the countries of heaviest immigration—Argentina, Uruguay, and Chile.

A more important difference refers to the timing of declines in the birth rate, since future population growth in Latin America will be much more affected by variation in fertility than in mortality. North American birth rates began declining at least from the beginning of the nineteenth century and continued to decline till 1940. In assessing future trends in Latin American fertility, therefore, it is important to keep in mind that it required about a century and a half for the United States to achieve birth rates comparable to those of Europe. (Most European countries, in turn, took at least this amount of time to bring their birth rates to modern levels.) It is usually argued that increasing urbanization, education, and income level will bring down birth rates soon in Latin America. Is there any reason to believe they will come down faster than they did in the United States?

First of all, we must not overlook the possibility that Latin American birth rates will *rise* before they begin to fall. This occurred in England and most Western European nations. In Latin America, there are several factors currently inhibiting fertility which might be expected to be reduced by economic modernization:

(1) Malnutrition or generally debilitating diseases which may impair fecundity or reduce the incidence of sexual relations will be reduced.

(2) Specific diseases such as gonorrhea which impair fecundity will be reduced.

(3) Relatively high ages at marriage in most Latin countries might be reduced by greater economic prosperity and security. Further, with increasing education and economic well-being, we may anticipate a reduction in consensual or "free" unions, which because of their unstable nature relative to marriage, are in some countries less fertile than legal unions.

(4) Breast feeding, which for some following a birth is as effective as a low-grade contraceptive, may decline in incidence or in duration with economic development.

Whether or not such changes would lead to an increase in the birth rate, depends upon the degree of counteracting practices such as abortion and contraception.

On the other hand, Argentina, Chile, and Uruguay have shown notable declines in birth rates in the past half century and may suggest an acceleration of the long process of fertility decline. A difficult question, however, is the extent to which such changes are due to changes in education and economic development, or to the European culture which characterizes these particular Latin American nations. Let us then look at the relation between fertility and economic and social development.

No one knows precisely how or why the birth rates of the United States and Western Europe were reduced, but a number of reasonable and partially confirmed hypotheses may be advanced:

(1) Reductions were accomplished largely by deliberate efforts to prevent conception or birth, rather than by changes in marriage pattern or declines in fecundity.

(2) Such efforts were brought about less by innovation in contraceptive technology than by broad social and economic changes which created strong penalties for high fertility.

(3) Fertility control spread from urban to rural areas, and from upper social classes to lower.

Since there is no reason to believe that changes in either age at marriage or in fecundity in Latin America will affect fertility negatively, let us proceed to the second point.

There is a basic difference between the control of death and the control of birth which must be kept in mind. Declines in the death rates of Europe and the United States took a great deal of time because they were probably less the result of medical technology than of gradual improvements in level of living, transportation, nutrition, and so on. These in turn were the result of broad social and economic changes. In short, the declines both in fertility and mortality stemmed from the general complex now referred to as "development" or "modernization."

In Latin America, on the other hand, declines in the death rate have been more rapid than was the case in North America and Europe, but not because economic development was more rapid. Indeed, the improvements in mortality occurred virtually independently of economic development because medical technology today, especially public health techniques, is so developed that mortality can be reduced without improving levels of living and education.

Can the same be said for control of fertility? There is no doubt that technological advances in contraception, making birth control easier, cheaper and more effective than in earlier periods, represent a potential factor in speeding the decline of fertility; but unlike death control, birth control is more likely to require social organizational changes which place penalties on having many children.

Among the changes believed to be associated with the intensification of such penalties are urbanization, industrialization, and education. While these topics receive detailed attention in subsequent chapters, it is relevant to note here that a fair amount of education, as much as five or six years, is required before a material impact on fertility occurs. For many countries it will be a long time before the general level of education reaches this stage. Urbanization in Latin America seems to be a different kind from that experienced by other countries where it was part of the industrialization process, possibly its consequence. Industrial growth has not kept pace with urbanization, and gains in non-agricultural activities are largely the result of increases in service occupations. Many migrants live in urban slums which will allow them to maintain much of their rural way of life. Whether urbanization of this kind will have a depressing effect on fertility is not known. Moreover, the gap between rural and urban areas in Latin America is far greater than has been the case in North America, and social class lines are more clearly maintained. Therefore, it may take longer for patterns of fertility control to permeate rural and lower-class groups. In short, there is some reason to doubt that fertility declines will be accelerated in Latin America without specific policies directed toward this goal.

There is nothing unique or intrinsically "wrong" with any single aspect of Latin America's demographic position. What is problematic and unusual is the combination of demographic facts: high fertility in the face of low mortality, rapid population increase and slow economic growth, urbanization without industrialization, low population density with agricultural overpopulation, and so on. It is the disequilibrium in these various aspects which causes difficulty and which begs for solution. It becomes more and more apparent that countries cannot avoid dealing in one way or another with population growth.

3

Latin American Intellectuals
and the Population Problem

Until very recently, North Americans tended to regard as unrealistic any suggestion of direct attack by Latin America on its population problem. The Catholic Church was viewed as the major stumbling block, due to the combination of its presumed hold over the consciences of 95 percent of Latin Americans, and its intransigence on the issue of population control. As it turns out, neither assumption had much validity. As we shall see, an increasing number of sample surveys in Latin American countries disclose that the average woman wants a moderate sized family, approves generally of family planning, and is little influenced by Church teaching on these topics. Further, the Church itself has shown increasing concern about the population problem and a willingness to discuss the morality of family planning. Indeed, the Church has had neither the need nor the inclination to do battle on this issue in Latin America, since most intellectuals were already opposed to population control for totally secular reasons. While clerical interest will do much to open up discussion of what a recent *Visión* editorial refers to as "the great tabu of our time," it will do little more; for the main opposition to *population control*, as opposed to family planning, continues to stem from Marxists, and from nationalists of the left and right.

An understanding of the viewpoints of these intellectuals is important both to avoid an excess of optimism over a possible liberalization of the Catholic position, and to give an appreciation of the nature of the real change in philosophy which is occurring in Latin America among the middle and upper classes.

DATA AND DEMOGRAPHERS

Before examining the opinion of intellectuals on demographic topics, we should have an idea of the amount and quality of demographic data which have been available to them, as well as of the status of demography as a scientific discipline in Latin America.

So European in many aspects, Latin America lagged behind Europe in developing a tradition of gathering systematic data through censuses and vital statistics. Only eight republics took population censuses between 1925 and 1934, and thirteen in the 1935–1944 period.[1] While virtually all nations took a census during the past ten years, Uruguay's recent census was its first in over half a century.

Data based on the registration of vital events are even more deficient. For example, only five of the twenty republics are considered to have reasonably complete registration of deaths, and these countries (Argentina, Chile, Costa Rica, El Salvador, and Mexico) account for only one-third of Latin America's population. Some of the reasons for the poor quality of birth and death registration are cited by Gaete-Darbó:

Registration is carried out by a large number of officials who work on a notably autonomous basis, separated from one another, with no possibility of consulting each other and with little advice or control; the statistical training of registration officials is practically nil . . . it is virtually sufficient to know how to read and write (in most countries) . . . in no country does training cover statistical work or scientific administration; registration of data depends partly on the registrar, partly on the community, and partly on the medical

[1] Giorgio Mortara, "Appraisal of Census Data for Latin America," *Milbank Memorial Fund Quarterly*, XLII (April 1964).

and paramedical group, . . . which makes it more complex, with errors in registration more difficult to discover and correct.[2]

As scarce as are good demographic statistics in Latin America, demographers to analyze them are even scarcer. "Despite the fact that most countries now take periodic censuses," notes one observer, "analysis of these data leaves much to be desired."[3] "Relatively few articles which appear in internationally read journals are written by Latin American scholars," writes another commentator. Even the official journal of the Inter-American Statistical Association, *Estadística*, "has had to fill its pages with translations because of the lack of original material."[4] As one measure of the professional contributions of Latin American demographers, we may look at the national origins of contributors to the World Population Conferences (see Table 1). At the first conference, held in Rome in 1954, 13 Brazilians presented papers, but the other 19 Latin American republics were represented by only a dozen contributors—only one more than the Netherlands delegation, and well under the number of readers of papers for either Japan or India. A decade later, at the Belgrade Conference, the number of Latin American contributors of papers had declined from 25 to 21 and the proportion of Latin American contributors from 7 to 4 percent. (These figures do not include contributions of Latins working in international organizations. At the 1965 meeting, there were contributions on Latin America by six members of the United Nations Latin American Demographic Center and four members of CEPAL.)

Another measure of the size of the profession is provided by

[2] A. Gaete-Darbó, "Appraisal of Vital Statistics in Latin America," *Milbank Memorial Fund Quarterly*, XLII (April 1964).

[3] Waldermiro Bazanella, "Areas de Prioridad en la Investigación Social en América Latina," in *Ciencias Políticas y Sociales*, XXVI (October 1961), p. 520.

[4] Nathan Keyfitz, "Assessment of Teaching and Training Program in the Universities of Latin America," *Milbank Memorial Fund Quarterly*, XLII (April 1964), 236–37.

Table 1. Place of origin of contributors of papers to World
Population Conferences, 1954 and 1965 (in percent)

Origin	1954	1965
Latin America	7	4
Africa	4	4
Asia	8	17
North America[a]	25	22
Eastern Europe (including USSR)	2	18
Western Europe and Oceania	44	21
International organizations[b]	10	14
Total	100	100
Number of contributors	(359)	(547)

[a] Includes English-speaking Caribbean and Puerto Rico.
[b] Since it was often difficult to establish the national origins of members
of international organizations, they were given a separate classification.

data on membership in the International Union for the Scientific
Study of Population. In 1964 Africa had 19 members, Asia 78,
the United States and Canada 143, and Europe 279. Latin America had only 49, of which Argentina, Brazil, and Chile accounted
for 31. Japan and the Netherlands each had almost twice as many
members as Mexico and Central America combined, while Japan
and India together had six more members than all of Spanish-
speaking Latin America.[5]

The situation with respect to training shows Latin Americans
similarly disadvantaged. Most fellowships for the graduate study
of demography are given by the Population Council. As shown
below, as many fellowships have gone to Koreans in the past ten
years as to citizens of the twenty Latin American republics.

But Population Council fellowships are normally for study in
the United States or Europe. What about training in Latin
America itself? The principal facility at the present time is the
Centro Latinoamericano de Demografía (CELADE) in Santiago,
Chile. Organized by the United Nations in 1957, the Center has

[5] Figures taken from *Le Démographe,* October 1964.

Table 2. Demographic fellowships,
the Population Council, 1953–1964

Africa	18
Asia (Total)	109
India	44
Pakistan	13
Japan	14
Korea	9
Other	29
Latin America	9

Source: Data in *The Population Council Newsletter*, March 1965.

offered instruction in technical aspects of demography to about fifteen students per year. There is general agreement among experts that the quality of instruction is very high, that staff and students are extremely hard working, that administration is efficient, and that morale is high. However, the impact of this institution on *national* development of demography in Latin America has been disappointing. Of the 89 students trained between 1958 and 1963 few came from or have risen to positions of influence in government or universities. Indeed, because of the quality and background of the students and the brief period of training, "only a rather small group," according to CELADE's director, "will eventually be demographers."[6] Only four graduates are now engaged in full-time teaching, although a dozen more may teach a course or two.

The absence of demographic teaching or research in Latin American universities is a key to the problem. CELADE cannot train people for positions which do not exist, nor can it attract high-quality academic students if they have never heard of demography. It has had to rely largely on governmental nominations of middle-level civil servants from official statistical bureaus.

[6] Carmen Miró, "Principles and Practices of Teaching and Training in CELADE," *Milbank Memorial Fund Quarterly*, XLII (April 1964), 219.

In the meantime few inroads have been made in the Latin American universities, the great majority of which offer not a single course in demography.

Even in Brazil where, because of the efforts of G. Mortara, a relatively distinguished tradition in demography has been established, Mortara could speak of the "contempt for demography in the organization of university programs." He noted wryly that in the faculties of statistical sciences there is only one course in demographic statistics and in the faculties of philosophy and economics "a half-course," and concludes that true development of scientific research in demography requires "a modification in higher education which would grant this discipline the place it merits among the course materials of economic, social and administrative sciences."[7]

It may seem strange that this demographic desert should exist in the universities of Latin America where, unlike most underdeveloped regions, academic institutions have been well entrenched for one or two centuries. Further, sociology and economics, the disciplines most intimately associated with demography in the United States and Europe, have long been recognized disciplines in Latin American universities. Sociology, the study of which began in the nineteenth century, now has hundreds of professorial chairs, and chairs of economics are even more numerous. Actually, the absence of demographic work in the universities is largely due to the peculiar development of the social sciences in Latin America, where sociology was early established along non-empirical, humanistic, and literary lines, strongly under the dominance of the powerful schools of law; and where economics was more allied to accounting and business administration than to science. While the scientifically inclined tended to enter technological professions such as medicine and engineering, "sociology" tended to be such an amorphous disci-

[7] G. Mortara, "Demographic Studies in Brazil," in P. Hauser and O. D. Duncan, *The Study of Population* (Chicago: Chicago University Press, 1959).

pline that "lawyers, literary men, and even physicians were called 'sociologists.' "[8] Indeed, the early acceptance and institutionalization of "sociology" has impeded its progress as a modern discipline in Latin America, and scientifically oriented schools or departments emerged in Latin American institutions only in the 1950's. Even now, however, only a minimal amount of demography is provided in the newer institutes,[9] partly because the field has been viewed as more appropriate for government technicians in the census bureaus or statistical services. At the moment, the only possibility for academic demographic study at the graduate level in a Latin American national institution is provided at the Centro de Estudios Demográficos y Económicos of the Colegio de México.

ATTITUDES TOWARD THE PROBLEM
OF POPULATION

The Pronatalist Position

In addition to the absence of adequate demographic data and the low status of demography as a scientific discipline, Latin Americans have long lived in a psychological atmosphere of *under*population. The Spanish and Portuguese settlers were acutely conscious of their small numbers vis à vis the Indians, who were often reluctant to work for the colonizers. At various periods and places different schemes were devised for obtaining a labor force sufficient to work the mines, the plantations, and the haciendas: the encomienda and mita systems and slavery were

[8] Orlando Fals Borda, "Desarrollo y Perspectivas de la Sociología Rural en Colombia y la América Latina," *Memorias del Primer Congreso Nacional de Sociología* (Bogotá: Editorial Iqueima, 1963).

[9] For an early discussion of courses see E. Dieulefait, "The Teaching of Demography in Latin America," *The University Teaching of Demography* (UNESCO, 1957).

efforts at providing cheap manpower, generally for rural pursuits. Later, a number of Latin American countries encouraged massive European immigration, just as did the United States and Canada. While the problem of scarce labor has been replaced by that of unemployment and underemployment in Latin America, the mystique of the rural frontier lives on, and Latins still speak longingly of peopling their wide-open spaces. Argentina's former Ambassador to the United Nations recently echoed this sense of manifest destiny: "If we are capable of creating together those opportunities, the next century will see more than five hundred million Latin Americans living prosperously, in order to fulfill the historic destiny that God has willed us."[10] Mixed in this statement, one can see elements of various beliefs—that people are power, that people are wealth, and that the Latin American people are noble. The belief that people are power is understandable in the light of the colonial psychology of the Spanish and Portuguese settlers, and even toward the end of the nineteenth century, Argentina's Juan Bautista Alberdi could pronounce the dictum "Gobernar es poblar." But a more frequently heard theme today is that people are wealth, in the sense of labor force and as a source of internal markets. In the case of a Brazilian Minister of Health it seems to be muscle power:

In underdeveloped countries such as Brazil, where over 50 percent of the energy utilized in production is muscular in nature, population size constitutes a real element of power which is the most important means of national progress. Therefore, anything which increases population growth is beneficial for us.[11]

But for others it means brain power. For Victor Belaúnde of Peru, unborn children are potential capital which must not go unexploited:

[10] Mario Amadeo, *Revista Claudia*, Buenos Aires, 1964.
[11] Speech at the World Health Organization, Geneva, March 1964.

39

Can we know the mystery of unborn men, who might have brought a new message for humanity? The greatest capital is the inventive genius of man.[12]

Mario Amadeo of Argentina and Rodríguez Fabregat of Uruguay combine the concepts of brain and muscle and see a plentitude of people as assuring both:

Italy and Holland, what is the source of their good fortune? Their populations—the alert mind and strong arm of their children.[13]

The newborn child should be regarded not as an extra mouth to feed, but as an additional mind and an additional pair of hands which could make a contribution to the progress of mankind.[14]

Finally, there is the population-as-goad school of thought, which holds that suffering and deprivation are useful or even necessary since they stimulate man to creative solutions. Mexicans, who have been generously endowed by these standards, have been especially articulate on the topic:

Demographic pressures create social and political forces which tend to accelerate progress and to show, with greater clarity, the characteristics and the gravity of these problems. Without these demographic pressures I consider that the progressive evolution of this world would be slower and I doubt that it would be less burdensome.[15]

[12] Report of the United Nations Population Commission, December 18, 1962 (mimeo.). We will draw frequently on unpublished United Nations documents summarizing committee meetings on the population question. In such documentation, speakers are normally paraphrased rather than directly quoted.

[13] Mario Amadeo, *op. cit.*

[14] Rodríguez Fabregat, Uruguayan delegate to the U.N. Population Commission, March 13, 1961.

[15] Gilberto Loyo, in *Problemas Demográficos de México*, cited in L. Nye Stevens, "Problems of Population Growth," *Public and International Affairs*, XI (Fall 1963), 121.

I believe that demographic pressures as in other countries have been a progressive factor in Mexico's economy. This pressure has to a great measure forced us to look for a better way to use our resources.[16]

With a very rapid demographic increase, year by year the standard of living rises—slowly, it must be admitted. This is because little exploited natural resources are important, and because the increase in density works in favor of economic progress.[17]

The Mexican stance in general is the prototype of the nationalistic pronatalist position. The following quotation, summarizing the attitudes of 120 well-educated Mexican males recently surveyed, shows the equation of population size with power, prestige, and dynamism:

Mexico was once weak, divided and helpless, her people were dominated by alien conquerors, and she was under-populated, her lands were taken by foreign invaders. But Mexico is growing. There is strength in numbers. True, numbers bring problems, but we are forging these numbers into a great nation.[18]

Indifference Toward the Population Problem

The most characteristic attitude toward population growth in Latin America is indifference. This is not surprising, since both population size and rate of growth have not been remarkable until recently. As late as 1920 the total population of the twenty republics of Latin America was less than the present population of Indonesia or Pakistan. With only about nine persons for every square kilometer, Latin America has a population density half

[16] Luis Velásquez Peña, *México*, cited in Arthur Corwin, *Contemporary Mexican Attitudes Toward Population, Poverty and Public Opinion* (Gainesville: University of Florida Press, 1963), p. 6.

[17] Rubio L. García, "El Desarrollo Demográfico de México y sus Exigencias Económico-Sociales," *Revista Internacional de Sociología*, XIV (1961), 561–562.

[18] Arthur Corwin, *op. cit.*, p. 42.

that of the United States and one-tenth that of Europe. As late as the period 1925–1935 only two countries had annual growth rates as high as 2.5 percent, whereas in the decade ahead (1965–1975) sixteen nations will fall in this category, with four of them growing at 3.5 percent or more.[19] The novelty of current rates of growth and the failure to distinguish problems of absolute size or density from problems of growth account for much of the indifference. In maintaining that there is no problem of population growth, however, one school of thought believes it literally, and another believes that the "population problem" is in fact something else. For the "literal school" the problem is quickly dismissed by references to density:

A demographic explosion is inconceivable in a continent of over 13,000,000 kilometers with a population in 1962 of about 226,000,000. ... It may seem to be premature and almost absurd to worry about the rapid increase in population, especially if it is remembered that there are many empty spaces in Latin America.[20]

... our Argentina, young, vigorous, and with surprising economic possibilities, with three million square kilometers and 20 million inhabitants; reducing the birth rate would be absurd.[21]

Despite its demographic evolution, Latin America does not face an immediate threat of over-population, since it has approximately a seventh part of the earth's surface, and only a tenth of its population.[22]

A second school of thought maintains that what seems like a population problem is in fact an economic or political problem. If a nation's wealth is not growing with sufficient speed, it is due to deficiencies in the productive and distributive sphere. Indeed,

[19] Growth data and estimates from C. Miró, "The Population of Latin America," *Demography*, 1, No. 1 (1964), Table 2, p. 17.

[20] *International Migration*, II, No. 1 (1964).

[21] Alfredo L. Palacios, *Revista Claudia, op. cit.*

[22] *El Tiempo* (Bogotá), April 10, 1963, reporting on the publication of the *U.N. World Social Situation* for 1963.

the "population problem" is not only fictitious but a deliberately created myth of the imperialist nations. The latter point of view has been a classical Marxist position, and was well expressed in the United Nations Population Commission by Mr. Solodovnikov, the delegate from the Soviet Union.

There had been references to a population explosion presenting a threat even more serious than nuclear weapons. Some Western circles were making use of those neo-Malthusian ideas to distract world public opinion from the real causes of the poverty of the underdeveloped countries, by attributing economic backwardness to excessively rapid population growth, rather than to long years of exploitation in the colonial era. Efforts were being made to use the United Nations to spread propaganda on the subject and to disseminate theories which were at variance with reality. The demographic problem was not in fact a real one. It existed only because in some countries the level of production was too low and was not rising at the same rate as the population. His delegation thought it was the duty of the United Nations bodies, and particularly of the Population Commission, to speak out against Malthusian explanations of population changes. If population problems were to be eliminated, emphasis must be placed on the development of all sectors of the economy of developing countries, particularly agricultural production, and on improved standards of living and education for the population, rather than on efforts to find ways of decreasing the population.[23]

Some representatives of this point of view feel that the admission of a population problem is so defeatist or pessimistic that they *refuse* to admit it. A population approach is viewed as "negative" or "static" rather than "positive" or "dynamic."

ATTITUDES TOWARD BIRTH CONTROL

The subject of birth control, the limitation of birth by voluntary means, can usefully be divided into two: population control,

[23] U.N. Population Commission, April 9, 1963.

the limitation of birth in order to slow the rate of growth of a nation or some other large collectivity; and family planning, which is birth control in the service of the health or well-being of the family. Espousal of one of these does not necessarily mean espousal of the other. In the United States the work of Margaret Sanger was almost entirely in the service of family planning, whereas more recently there are organizations which concentrate on population control. (An interesting coalition of these two camps was formed recently under the title of the Planned Parenthood Federation of America-World Emergency Campaign.) It will be necessary to examine the attitudes toward each of these aspects of birth control.

Attitudes Toward Population Control

In a public lecture a few years ago the Mexican economist and demographer Gilberto Loyo stated that "in all other matters we are planners, but in matters of population we are still *laissez faire.*"[24] Latins who take this position are not saying that population is not a problem—they are saying that they are unwilling to do anything about it. Víctor Urquidi washed his hands of it in this way:

Fundamentally, population control is a cultural problem. I am an economist, I don't believe it is a problem for an economist. A demographic growth rate of 3 percent is a fact. I accept it. This means we simply have to plan the economy taking this fact into account.[25]

If the economists refuse to deal with the problem, what about the physicians? On the whole, they do the same. Many physicians express themselves as did Dr. José Álvarez Amezquita, Mexico's Secretary of Health, when he rejected birth control by explaining that "the physician is always for life and against death."[26] If the physician's job is to save life and not to stop it, then he can

[24] Corwin, *op. cit.,* p. 2.   [25] *Ibid.*
[26] *La Prensa* (Mexico City), August 16, 1963.

virtually measure his success by the increasing population. If it is pointed out that this is causing economic problems, many physicians reply, "Then let the economists solve it." The net result of the physicians' and economists' refusal to tackle the problem was, as late as 1963, that

none of the Latin American countries have even considered the adoption of a policy aimed at slowing down the rate of population increase. . . . The continuation of high rates of increase is therefore taken for granted in development plans.[27]

According to a prevalent view in Latin America, while population influences other things, it must not or cannot be influenced by deliberate means. It is regarded as an "independent variable," acting on other dependent variables. But why does it have this unique nature? In an age when economic planners determine who and how many shall be educated, what crops will be produced by whom, and how sickness should be treated, why should the rate of population growth not be a variable to be influenced rather than be a "given"?

For some, economic development is a *means*, population an *end*. To tamper with the latter for the benefit of the former seems a perversion. Mr. Temboury, then Spanish delegate to the United Nations Population Commission, expressed it in the following terms:

Economic development should serve mankind and raise the level of living of all human beings. The resolution before the Committee (technical assistance on population) had inverted the relationship and would make man subservient to economic development.[28]

The Uruguayan delegate objected to the statement that "each government must decide for itself whether or not any measures should be taken for the purpose of modifying the trends of

[27] *1963 U.N. Report on the World Social Situation*, p. 123.
[28] U.N. Population Commission, December 12, 1962.

population," feeling that demographic trends should not be modified: "The solution was to improve economic conditions rather than to allow them to dictate what the size of the population should be."[29]

To talk of population is to conjure up images of life itself, with all its mysteries. Should we attempt to bring science and control over such a sacred area? "How is it possible," writes a Colombian columnist, "that science finds itself incapable of giving a more human solution, something less cruel than stopping the fountains of life?"[30]

Victor Belaúnde also raised this question in the United Nations:

Albert Schweitzer . . . has said that life is something sacred. Life, moreover, is a great mystery, and all aspects of origin, development, obstacles and manifestations of life must be dealt with with the greatest of care. . . . Do we know that moral consequences may flow from measures taken to limit the population, measures which assume the exercise of biological functions without the responsibility, not even the moral responsibility of procreation and the necessity of caring for one's progeny? . . . Everybody here knows that certain movements which promote genetic control brought about the decline of civilization.[31]

Thus, when we interfere with life's mysteries it can have unknown evil consequences in the moral or genetic sphere. There is also the lurking fear of *state* control over the most intimate aspects of life—a control which could lead to especially nefarious abuses:

If birth control were to be admitted, it would only be a matter of time before such monstrous practices as abortion, "mercy" killing and the destruction of the old were accepted.[32]

[29] Rodríguez Fabregat, U.N. Population Commission, March 13, 1961.
[30] Rosa Margarita Puccini, *El Espectador* (Colombia), July 8, 1964.
[31] U.N. Population Commission, December 18, 1962.
[32] Temboury, U.N. Population Commission, December 12, 1962.

In Puerto Rico . . . the policy of birth control had produced only insignificant results. That was why various specialists no longer hesitated to propose measures of compulsory sterilization. It was possible to see how far certain theories based on a misconception of the determinants of economic development could lead.[33]

Combined with the fear of tampering, especially the state's tampering with human life, is the idea that to *let nature take its course* with respect to population will result in automatic solution of the problem. If the problem will take care of itself why worry about it? It is felt that the process of industrialization and education will inevitably bring about fertility declines. Since Latin American countries are doing everything possible to educate their population and to industrialize their cities, they are doing as much as is necessary to take care of the population problem.

The rational control of birth as a product of culture, not its cause . . . as a society industrializes, increases its literary level, and urbanizes, . . . almost automatically births are diminished.[34]

Arguments in favor of direct action on conception do not take into account the teachings of the demographic history of the whole world. . . . If this rate of urbanization persists in Mexico it will necessarily result in a diminution of general fecundity.[35]

There is something about this "spontaneous" process of reducing fertility that is superior to the "artificial" process of encouraging population control. Indeed, on occasion the writers seem to forget that industrialization and education cannot directly affect natality, but must do so precisely through such means as birth control.

The real way (to establish) a new vital balance in those countries will never be the directed control of births, but rather the utiliza-

[33] Bernardo, Argentine delegate to U.N. Population Commission, December 19, 1962.
[34] Pangloss, *El Espectador* (Colombia), July 6, 1964.
[35] R. Benítez Zenteno, cited in N. Stevens, *op. cit.,* p. 126-27.

tion of the instruments of economic and social transformation which create conditions for the spontaneous reduction of birth rates.[36]

The mean rate of population growth in Argentina—the lowest in Latin America—was the outcome not of a policy of birth control or of dissemination of neo-Malthusian practices, but of the effects of industrialization and the concentration of the population in the towns.[37]

Beneath many of these fears of interference with nature, or of "control," lies a lurking fear that population control is an instrument of the imperialists for emasculating or at least controlling peoples of the underdeveloped areas—especially those of another color: what else could account for what appears to many Latin Americans as the Yankee obsession for the control of population in *other* countries?

A characteristic of this school (neo-Malthusianism) which is deeply resented by the peoples of underdeveloped countries, is that it invariably and single-mindedly proposes limitation of births. They are concerned about reducing the number of Puerto Ricans, Hindus, Negroes, Chinese and Mexicans; or else, of certain classes and social groups, like the poor, the working class, or the Catholics. But they do not worry, for example, about the increase of Aryans, of Protestants, or of Rotarians.[38]

Attitudes Toward Family Planning

Quite apart from the question of population control is birth control for the welfare of the family unit. The school of thought which regards family planning positively cites various advantages to the family of moderate size: health of the mother, psychological benefits through freedom from fear of unwanted pregnancies and from unwanted children, superior per capita

[36] Wilson Fadul, *Brazil*, March 10, 1963.
[37] Bernardo, Argentine delegate to the U.N. Population Commission, December 19, 1962.
[38] E. Flores, cited in N. Stevens, *op. cit.*, p. 118.

socialization of the children, greater opportunities for personal and social development of the parents, and the like.

Those taking a negative point of view toward family planning less frequently contest these advantages than allege various kinds of social, psychological, moral, and physical side effects which accompany mechanical, chemical, or surgical means of family planning.

A full range of medical and psychiatric arguments has also been raised against birth control. The recent statement by the Mexican gynecologist Dr. Alfonso Álavarez Bravo is typical in its scope:

No contraceptive method is harmless. On the contrary, the use of these methods will aggravate existing pathological conditions. In not a few cases, such methods provoke individual intolerances, predispose to the appearance and development of cancer, cause changes in the endocrine glands, the hypophysis, and in the female reproductive organs, and can likewise diminish future fertility and even inhibit fertility forever. . . . The psychic disturbances produced by the contraceptives form a sober gamut of frustration and disturbing inhibitions, guilt complexes, especially in religious persons.[39]

A Case Example

As a way of summarizing the various points of view in favor of rapidly increasing population and against population control, let us consider the many-sided articulations of a single individual. An influential and dedicated writer, the editor of San Salvador's *El Diario de Hoy*, N. Viera Altamirano, has been one of the most vociferous exponents of a Latin America massive in numbers. To Altamirano population is almost a mystical force, and Latin America's destiny lies in its population growth. "To populate America is to civilize America," he wrote in 1962. "To oppose population is to oppose civilization."[40]

[39] *Excelsior* (Mexico City), May 14, 1964.
[40] *El Diario de Hoy* (San Salvador), January 25, 1962.

Altamirano is fairly specific about the population he considers desirable. He speaks longingly of Central America's being a truly great nation like England, France, or Japan, and says it should think of birth control only after it has twice the population of England or France. At one point he speaks of Central America's resources being sufficient for a population ten times its present size, and elsewhere maintains that Latin America as a whole needs "two billion more inhabitants to reach the optimal level."[41] A problematic size might be reached only when "the rest of Latin America has reached a population of at least four billion."[42]

Altamirano's nationalism is closely linked to a racial mystique. Through his writing it is clear that he views the Indian, the Mestizo, and the person of color to be the "authentic" Latin. Since he would like to see Latins increase and multiply themselves from ten to twenty times, any talk of population control is viewed as "discrete genocide," "the new cannibalism," and a "racist conspiracy." The conspiracy is apparently not limited to foreigners, however, for he refers to "married couples who from the first day conspire against the race. We regard this as the new opiate of civilization."[43]

The North Americans and Europeans are extremely concerned over the growth of the colored population in the nations of America, Africa, Asia, and Australia.[44]

... the conspiracy against the colored races, and especially against the Spanish American peoples, in the form of a new neo-Malthusianism which will end in birth control.[45]

We should not allow them to come from outside to sterilize the wombs of the hispanic-american mothers, whether they be negroes, mestizos, creoles or cobrizas.[46]

[41] *Ibid.*   [42] *El Diario de Hoy*, March 18, 1963.
[43] *Ibid.*, November 11, 1962.   [44] *Ibid.*, March 18, 1963.
[45] *Ibid.*, June 21, 1963.   [46] *Ibid.*, January 25, 1962.

White nations are growing rich in people and wealth, at the expense both of number of people and wealth of "their adversaries."

The white European will be proud of his intelligence, because he will have stopped the growth of his adversaries, while he has achieved an immense population. . . . [Europe] can continue counting on raw materials which permit her to grow without the necessity of spending her resources.[47]

From sterilization, Altamirano soon passes to other horrors. Birth control is listed in one editorial as the modern parallel of slave trade, opium traffic, and head-hunting. In another he likens it to malaria, hook worm, syphilis, morphine, and alcohol in slowing the march of civilization. One editorial entitled "The Beheading of the Holy Innocents" suggests that the arrival of birth control to Latin America will be another Herodean massacre of the innocents. Apparently captured by this analogy, he weaves it into his concern that the wombs of Latin women will be sliced by Malthusian knives:

These concerned birth controllers, whose racist interest can be divined on inspection, come to us speaking of the end of the world, with the gentle face of preachers, but concealing behind their backs the knife of Herod . . . in order to stop in the very womb of the Latin mother the impetuous current of the life created by Providence.[48]

Altamirano's editorials display a certain scorn for Keynesian economics, agrarian reform, and socialism. Apparently opposed to planning in the economic sphere, he is doubly opposed to it in the family sphere. On occasion he will employ phrases as "la familia dirigida," "la familia regimentada," or even "la vida dirigida" as synonyms for birth control. From here it is a short

[47] *Ibid.*, October 22, 1962.
[48] *Ibid.*, May 18, 1963.

literary step to the antiseptic family devoid of love or mystery, a kind of scientific rabbit hutch promoted by the imperialist nation in order to keep the colonies under control. Ultimately, we have created the human automaton of the totalitarian state.

All that remains is for them to set up matrimonial courses in which the future parents can plan not only the number of children . . . but their sex and character as well.[49]

. . . directed, planned family . . . aseptic, molded like cattle, like apiculture and aviculture. Above all so that the colored population, regimented and ordered, will never worry the old countries.[50]

In (China and Russia) all the totalitarian abuses will culminate with the planned family, the regimented family, the child to be born or not according to the State's decennial plans. Regimentation from conception to burial will have been accomplished.[51]

Altamirano's most comprehensive burst occurred as part of an attack on the World Food and Agricultural Congress. In a few lines he recapitulated his arguments of manifest destiny, nationalism, anti-imperialism, antisocialism, and genocide:

. . . the influence of true conspirators against our America, who come with a plan of massive destruction! The plan to destroy the capital of Latin America, to frighten away private investment, to socialize us before we have capitalized, and to block our growth cutting the womb of Latin mothers, castrating Latin males, before our peoples have grown sufficiently or taken possession of the vast empty lands of the continent.[52]

But Altamirano blends his deepest political and sexual fears in the following succinct statement: "We would say that the password for our Latin America is socialize and castrate her."[53]

[49] *Ibid.*, November 11, 1962.   [50] *La Prensa Libre* (San José).
[51] *Diario de Hoy*, October 22, 1962.   [52] *Ibid.*, June 21, 1963.
[53] *La Prensa Libre* (San José).

LATIN AMERICAN GOVERNMENTS AND BIRTH CONTROL

Official government policies on population control or family planning are only just emerging in Latin America, but on at least two occasions within recent times governments have had an opportunity to take a position. On the first occasion, a decade ago, legislation was proposed at the World Health Organization (WHO) to permit technical assistance on family planning to nations desiring it. According to the testimony of participants, the issue nearly tore WHO apart, and several Latin American countries threatened to resign if the matter were even discussed. A coalition of Communist and Catholic countries defeated the resolution, and, as far as can be determined, no Latin American country supported it.

In 1962 the governments were again presented an opportunity to vote for this kind of proposition, this time in the United Nations. Twelve African, European, and Asian nations sponsored a resolution to the General Assembly on "Population Growth and Economic Development." The final amended resolution was approved in the General Assembly with no negative votes, but by this time had lost its most important item, Article 6, which stated that the "United Nations give technical assistance, as requested by Governments, for national projects and programs dealing with problems of population." This article was singled out for special voting both in a preliminary review committee of the whole (where it was passed) and in the General Assembly (where it was rejected). Table 3 shows the distribution by geographic regions of the General Assembly vote.

While Latin America was the region most opposed to the technical assistance clause, the nations were by no means unanimous in their opposition. Since the pattern of voting in the review

Table 3. Distribution of General Assembly vote on Article 6, 1962, by geographic regions (in percent)

Vote	Asia	North America, Europe, and Oceania	Africa	Latin America
In favor	42	38	41	14
Abstained	50	28	26	24
Opposed	8	34	33	62
Total	100	100	100	100
No. of countries	(24)	(29)	(27)	(21)

committee (usually by different delegates from those in the General Assembly) gives us an additional indication of the predisposition of Latin American nations on the subject of population problems and control, we have made a classification of countries from most to least favorable to population control based on (1) sponsorship of the original resolution; (2) voting in the Second Committee for the resolution including Article 6, and (3) voting in the General Assembly on Article 6. In a few cases of unusual combinations, weight has been given to the General Assembly vote.

While there is a clear tendency in the negative direction, a fair range of attitudes is evidenced. Although no Latin American nation sponsored the original resolution, Chile and Costa Rica voted in favor of Technical Assistance both in the General Assembly and in Committee, whereas Argentina, Colombia, Perú and Uruguay consistently voted against. Most countries fell somewhere in between.

The General Assembly finally passed a revised resolution requesting the Secretary General to conduct an inquiry on population problems and economic development among the member governments. An extensive questionnaire was sent out, but by the time of the Secretary General's report in November 1964, only six Latin American nations had replied. Of these, Bolivia was uncommitted on the question of the relation of population

Category	Latin American Countries
1. Most favorable to population control: Sponsors of original resolution	None
2. Voted in favor of resolution in committee and of Article 6 in General Assembly	Chile Costa Rica
3. Abstained both in committee and in General Assembly	Cuba Haiti* Mexico Nicaragua* Panama
4. Abstained in committee; voted negatively in General Assembly	Bolivia Brazil Dom. Republic† Ecuador El Salvador Honduras† Paraguay† Venezuela
5. Voted negatively in committee and in General Assembly	Argentina Colombia Peru Uruguay

* Haiti voted positively and Nicaragua was not present in committee.
† The Dominican Republic and Paraguay did not vote, and Honduras voted positively in committee.

growth and economic development, Colombia and Guatemala merely observed that economic development has been too slow for the population growth rate, and Venezuela "views population growth, on the whole, as a positive factor in the development of the economy."[54] Certainly by the end of 1964, to judge by official positions, there seemed to be little reason for revising the

[54] U.N. Economic and Social Council, *Inquiry Among Governments on Problems Resulting from the Interaction of Economic Development and Population Changes*, 64-26191, November 1964.

conclusions of an earlier United Nations report which stated that "most of the countries look on the prospect of a population much larger than the present as a challenge, but not as a burden."[55]

As we shall see from other evidence in this volume, the foregoing analysis fails to take into account two important countervailing tendencies: the mounting concern in the 1960's among Latin American intellectuals that both economic and social progress were being threatened by excessively high rates of population growth, and the increasing interest of the general public in solution to the problem of growing family size. By the early 1970's many of the positions expressed here may be of only historical interest. In the early 1960's, however, they still dominated the official intellectual scene.

[55] *1963 U.N. Report on the World Social Situation*, p. 123.

II

ATTITUDES TOWARD
FAMILY SIZE AND
FAMILY PLANNING

4

Social Research on Fertility Control

Demographers spend most of their time correcting other people's mistakes. Traditionally the demographer has had little to say about the way in which his raw material—census data and birth and death registration data—is collected. Indeed, the data he uses are rarely collected with his interests in mind, but rather serve political, legal, or economic functions. As a result, the demographer has become especially skilled at correcting, adjusting, and twisting often fairly unreliable or deficient data to suit his purposes. While having very salutary consequences for the development of demographic methodology, this emphasis has tended to shift attention away from theory, and has limited the demographer's success in one of his most important activities, population forecasting.

Thus, in forecasting fertility, demographers have leaned heavily on elegant but mechanical extrapolations, which have not taken into account changes in human motivations. Human motivations have essentially fallen outside the demographer's analytic system, and the "soft data" of the social researcher have been regarded with somewhat condescending suspicion.

Furthermore, so strong have been our puritanical traditions about sex, that social scientists also neglected this area, leaving it to psychological investigators of the abnormal. Indeed it took a zoologist, Alfred Kinsey, to demonstrate to social scientists that mass collection of interview data on sexual behavior was feasible and reasonably reliable. But Kinsey's lesson did not come in time to affect the first social survey on fertility of a significant cross section of the American population—the Indianapolis Study of 1941. Despite batteries of questions and scores of psychological hypotheses, the study systematically avoided any questions of sex beyond contraception and fertility. Nevertheless, despite its failure to account for differential fertility or family planning, it too demonstrated that interviewing random samples of families on fertility behavior and attitude is no more difficult and no less reliable than social surveys on other topics.

The first major fertility survey conducted outside the continental United States was initiated less than two decades ago. Indeed, this survey, conducted by Paul Hatt in Puerto Rico in 1948, was probably the first representative sample of a total society with respect to fertility.[1] The interview contained a fertility and marital history of the female, and numerous questions of opinion, but the data on birth control and sexual relations were considered so unreliable that they were never reported.

In 1950, feeling that these limitations could be overcome by more intensive interviewer training, and desiring more extensive materials on the relation of sexual behavior to family planning, the writer initiated a "depth study" of seventy-two Puerto Rican families. Highly trained interviewers, using flexible techniques, interviewed lower-class couples for four to six hours on a wide range of topics potentially relevant to fertility.[2] (See Chapter 5.)

This study was followed by a series of Caribbean investigations throughout the fifties, ranging from highly qualitative projective approaches to standard survey methods applied to the subject of human fertility.[3] Various selections from these investi-

[1] P. K. Hatt, *Backgrounds of Human Fertility in Puerto Rico* (Princeton: Princeton University Press, 1952).

[2] J. M. Stycos, *Family and Fertility in Puerto Rico* (New York: Columbia University Press, 1955).

[3] R. Hill, J. M. Stycos, and K. W. Back, *The Family and Population Control* (Chapel Hill: University of North Carolina Press, 1959); J. Blake with J. M. Stycos and K. Davis, *Family Structure in Jamaica* (Glencoe, Ill.: Free Press, 1961); J. M. Stycos and K. W. Back, *The Control of Human Fertility in Jamaica* (Ithaca, N.Y.: Cornell University

gations are included in this part of the volume. Also throughout the fifties, investigators in the United States were beginning to apply survey methods to the study of fertility, so that by the end of the decade a landmark was reached when Whelpton's population projections included American couples' *intentions* about family size.[4]

By this time several surveys had been conducted in a number of Middle and Far Eastern countries, and had become common enough to be referred to by demographers as KAP surveys— surveys of knowledge, attitude, and practice relevant to family planning.

In the early 1960's, the writer initiated a KAP type survey in several Peruvian communities (see Chapters 10 and 15), the United Nations Demographic Center in Chile (CELADE) completed a survey for the city of Santiago de Chile,[5] and R. Benitez conducted a survey in Mexico City. Since none of these studies had profited from the experiences or designs of the others, Carmen Miró, Director of CELADE, and I decided that the time was ripe to do a series of fertility surveys employing comparable samples, questionnaires, and design. CELADE personnel visited a number of countries and elicited sufficient interest to launch, in collaboration with the International Population Program at Cornell University, the following proposal: KAP surveys would be carried out more or less simultaneously in each major city of an important group of countries. In each city representative samples of about 2,000 women in the reproductive age group would be systematically questioned. Personal interviews would be conducted, employing a basic questionnaire devised by the CELADE

Press, 1964); J. M. Stycos, "Haitian Attitudes Toward Family Size," *Human Organization*, XXIII (Spring 1964).

[4] R. Freedman, P. K. Whelpton, and A. A. Campbell, *Family Planning, Sterility and Population Growth* (New York: McGraw-Hill, 1959).

[5] L. Tabah and R. Samuel, "Preliminary Findings of a Survey of Fertility and Attitudes Toward Family Formation in Santiago, Chile," in C. V. Kiser, ed., *Research in Family Planning* (Princeton: Princeton University Press, 1962).

and Cornell staffs. The plan required a sponsoring institution in each nation, and a full-time local survey director attached to that institution.

Seven countries participated: Argentina, Brazil, Colombia, Costa Rica, Mexico, Panama, and Venezuela. (Peru and Chile were not included because similar studies had already been conducted there.) The sponsoring institutions included universities, international organizations, national statistical agencies, and combinations of these. Funds were provided by the Population Council, and during the summer of 1963 a training seminar for the study directors was held in Santiago. At that time U.N., Cornell, and CELADE personnel designed the questionnaire, instructed the group in sampling techniques, demonstrated interviewer-training techniques, pretested the questionnaire, and had members of the seminar do hand tallies of the ensuing data. The interview included a fertility history and questions relating to knowledge of and attitudes toward population growth, fertility, and contraception. Chapter 11 in the present volume contains some of the initial analyses of these data. More extensive reports are planned by CELADE, which is also initiating KAP-type surveys in *rural* areas of a number of Latin American countries. Aside from the scientific analyses which are made possible by the collection of such data, what are the functions of these surveys?

(1) They serve the cause of social science generally by demonstrating that social and psychological facts can be collected and interpreted scientifically. While any successful social survey might do the same, the KAP survey is especially effective because it deals with subject matter generally believed accessible only within the confessional. Thus it is a dramatic demonstration of the scope and flexibility of the social survey. In country after country we have been told, "It can't be done here. Our people will not answer such questions." Of course, when it *is* done, there is considerable incredulity: "Yes, they answer your questions, but did they tell the truth?" For this reason it is especially important to build in reliability and validity checks.

(2) The most important function of such surveys is similar to any market research project: to demonstrate the existence of a demand for goods or services, in this case for birth control. This may seem unnecessary or irrelevant in underdeveloped areas where excessive childbearing is only too obvious. But the elite in most societies believe that their people have many children because they want many children. They believe that there are deep-seated psychological motives to demonstrate fertility, pervasive cultural and religious norms to encourage maximum childbearing, and obsessive sexual and economic drives toward the production of a large family. They believe that to run counter to such a profound array of beliefs, drives, behavior patterns, and norms would either be political suicide or a waste of time. And indeed they would be correct if such assumptions were true. But, as we will see, the surveys demonstrate that couples want a moderate number of children, that they are convinced of the economic disadvantages of a large family, and that they are eager for information on what to do about it. Such information, if believed, can show that a program of population control could win votes rather than lose them.

(3) A third function of such studies relates to the fact that research is a relatively uncontroversial way of initiating activity in population control, in countries where direct efforts are not possible. The research itself, in addition to providing valuable information for possible future programs, stimulates the interest of those directly and indirectly involved, and may serve to accelerate the whole process of policy formation.

In Jamaica, for example, where a narrow balance of power existed in the 1950's between two political parties, both parties were unwilling to sponsor a population-control program for fear the opposition would use it against them; but it was possible to get agreement on action-oriented research, and to form a sponsoring board for the research that included representation from both sides.

In Latin America, the liberal wing of the Church is most eager to do something about the population problem, but, in the face of a negative, or at best unclear, position on the part of high Church authorities, it is naturally reluctant to engage in direct programs. Research, however, is permissible, and several Catholic institutions are about to embark on programs that go beyond KAP-type surveys and actually include contraceptive advice as part of the research design.

On the other hand, research can be used to delay action. A highly placed adviser of the Jamaican government publicly accused our Jamaican research project of holding up action on the part of the government. It got them off the hook, he charged, by letting them say, "Let's wait until all the facts are in." Undoubtedly, many a Latin American bishop over the next decade will be delighted to turn the problem of population increase over to Church scientists to investigate, so that a difficult decision can be postponed. But if the authorities are so ambivalent about action, the additional delay occasioned by such research is more than compensated for by the utility of the data provided. In other words, where commitment is weak it is especially important to have a structurally sound program.

(4) Finally, in terms of programming, such studies are valuable for indicating the kind of content which a family planning program might have. Are there important regional differences within a country which would affect content, or can the same type of program be applied throughout the nation? Are there differences between social classes, men and women, ethnic groups, young and old, which should be taken into account in programming? What are the areas of knowledge and ignorance about sexual matters and contraception which must be considered? How do present customs with respect to marriage, child-bearing, and child rearing affect fertility, and how could a program capitalize on such customs? These are among the many practical questions which KAP surveys can help to answer.

Most of the articles in this volume analyze demographic or

survey data less from the programmatic point of view than for their interest to social scientists and demographers generally. The program-oriented reader, however, should be able to see various implications for applied programs of fertility control.

5

Birth Control Clinics
in Crowded Puerto Rico

When the United States took possession of Puerto Rico at the turn of this century, the island had fewer than a million inhabitants; by 1950, with scant natural resources and a per capita income half that of Mississippi, its population had increased to more than two and a quarter million, despite heavy emigration. Only about half the land is arable, and the present number of people per square mile is roughly fifteen times that of the United States.

The increase in population has been brought about by spectacular declines in mortality, largely as a result of effective public health work. At the turn of the century, births were occurring annually at the rate of 40 per thousand, and deaths at the rate of about 25 per thousand, creating a relatively modest rate of increase. By mid-century the birth rate was still around 40—twice that of the United States—but the death rate had dropped to 10, roughly that of the continental United States. At this rate of increase, assuming no migration, the island would have approximately nine million inhabitants in another fifty years.

Aware that the island's program of development and industrialization was being undermined by a too rapidly expanding population, the government of Puerto Rico set up, in 1939, a network of 160 birth control clinics. Part of the extensive facilities of insular public health, these clinics are staffed by regular members of public health units, provided with contraceptives, and empowered to provide both information and free materials to all individuals who meet broadly interpreted medical criteria. The clinics carry condoms, diaphragms, creams, jellies, and sponges; are open for an afternoon or two a week; and are well located in both rural and urban areas of the small island. Despite this seemingly ideal setup, the clinics have as yet had no significant effect on the birth rate. In the first place, they are not used by most of the population—in 1950 the clinics showed 15,410 active cases—nor do the statistics over the past decade indicate any strong trend toward increasing use. Second, as we will explain, even those who acquire materials from the clinics do not use them systematically and carefully.

Why do the Puerto Ricans fail to take advantage of these readily available services, in light of the fact that more effective birth control would help substantially to relieve evident and pressing difficulties?

THE SITUATION

The Human Factors behind Resistance to Birth Control

A research project designed in part to discover the reasons for the ineffectiveness of the clinics was set up in 1951, under the auspices of the Family Life Project, Social Science Research Center, University of Puerto Rico. Seventy-two couples in the lower-income groups were interviewed on courtship, marriage, child rearing, and birth control. Husband interviews consumed about two hours, and wife interviews about four. Interviews were conducted by Puerto Ricans with academic and professional backgrounds in the social sciences and social work. Four women and two men were intensively trained in depth interviewing techniques for two weeks prior to field work. Using a flexible interview form, the team took verbatim notes in the presence of the respondents.

The following sections will summarize the factors found to

underlie the Puerto Ricans' reluctance to use the services of the birth control clinics. The findings fall into three general categories: attitudes toward family size, explicit and implicit objections to birth control practice, and the communication of birth control information.

Large Families or Small

An obvious reason for the Puerto Ricans' failure to use birth control would be that they are not interested in small families. If this were so, the public health program would have little effect unless accompanied by an educational campaign to stir up interest in smaller families. There is, however, evidence of some interest in reducing family size. In a 1948 poll of 13,000 randomly selected Puerto Ricans, over three-quarters of those interviewed stated that a family of three or fewer children is ideal. The writer's own case studies of seventy-two lower-class families reveal a similar interest in small families. Here are the remarks of a mother with two years of schooling:

If one is poor he shouldn't have more than two children. The rich can have more because they have money to educate them and do not sacrifice or even kill themselves working as the poor do. For the rich, they are even a recreation; for the poor man they are always a burden. The rich care better for the children, but it's a great task for the poor; and the wife of the poor man gets sick with many children, because she can't feed herself well nor have the proper medicines if she needs them. So two is enough.

Such attitudes are common. Parents feel that it is a burden to have many children; it requires hard work; it is a drain on family finances; and it is felt to be detrimental to health. This is not to say that children are not appreciated, for they are regarded with affection. It indicates rather that there is a growing awareness of the disadvantages of having a large number of children.

Evidently, then, there does exist sentiment in favor of small families. Other motivations, however, serve to foster the continuance of large families. For example, Puerto Ricans still say that children can help them in their old age, and that having a lot of children is a kind of social security that will pay dividends in later years. There is much less basis for this belief today than formerly, but many Puerto Ricans continue to believe it, or want to believe it—and the belief runs counter to the expressed desire for small families.

Again, while nearly everyone claims to want a small family, hardly anyone thinks of delaying the first pregnancy. One reason for this is the male fear of sterility. Lower-class Puerto Rican men are very conscious of their virility, and try to manifest it in different ways. One way is having children, and a married man without children is laughed at. Although men ordinarily have sexual experiences before marriage, these encounters are usually with prostitutes. Only by marrying and having children can men give manifest "proof" of virility. Most of the men in our sample said they were eager to have their first child. These are some of their explanations:

A man feels more man when he knows he can make a child.

I was anxious to have my first child to see if I was sterile or not, because one has to avoid children with other women before marriage.

This business of being married and having no children looks bad. One likes to have them to prove he is not barren.

Having a child is also a kind of initiation into the community of adults. Without children, a man is still a youth, or worse, only half a man.

My brother-in-law, who is only sixteen, got married, had a child, and his wife is now pregnant again. When he fights with other men people tell him he is not a man, he is only sixteen. But he tells them, "Well, I have children, I am a complete man."

As in many cultures where the double standard of sexual behavior prevails, men are extremely jealous of their wives, and wives are very unsure and suspicious of their husbands. There is some realistic justification for these feelings, for there is in fact a great deal of desertion and extramarital activity. Even so, the emotional reaction to such occurrences is unusually intense. These strong sentiments have an effect on attitudes toward family size. There are both men and women who feel that having a large number of children ties down their spouses and helps to keep them faithful. This technique works better for holding a woman than a man, but the illustrations below show that women as well as men are well aware of it.

He told me the more kids I have the more tied to him I was . . . that with so many kids I could not abandon him to go with another man or return to my family.

By having children they know that their wives are obliged to stay at home while they can go out after other women.

In one case this policy was carried out quite methodically. The story was told independently by both husband and wife. The husband told the interviewer that he had wanted no children at all and was then asked why he had just had one.

Because I got angry with my wife. Her mother took her to town and got her work as a servant. Later she came back to me full of love, and I forgave her so she stopped working. I had that child so that she couldn't go away any more. Having a child she was bound to stay.

Thus, even though individuals say they prefer small families, there are other forces operative in Puerto Rican culture that work at cross-purposes. Along with the expressed preference for small families one finds attitudes, beliefs, and practices that support the traditional custom of having large families.

Objection to Birth Control

Birth control and the Church. As in other Catholic countries, the church in Puerto Rico officially opposes birth control. However, most people do not regard church opposition as a reason for not controlling family size. In the extensive survey conducted by Paul Hatt, 87 percent of those interviewed claimed the right to limit family size if they so wished; other studies in Puerto Rico showed that specifically religious reasons for not practicing birth control are those least frequently cited. For the Puerto Rican lower classes Catholicism is in considerable part a series of rituals that are combined with social festivals, and a cult of saints to bring good fortune. People are aware of the attitude of the Church, but many tend to disregard it.

The Catholic religion says it's a sin to use birth control, but I think it's a greater sin if (the children) don't eat.

The Church forbids birth control, but if one has many children the church is not going to support them.

Our own survey showed that the few respondents who did cite church opposition as a reason for objecting to birth control were those with the smallest families; they had not yet felt any real need for birth control practice. Church opposition has even served to foster interest in birth control:

A pastoral letter, read in all the churches in one region, denouncing a newly established mountain clinic which had performed a number of sterilizations, generated most effective word-of-mouth advertising. . . . The clinic was swamped with demands for information concerning the operation which the Bishop had denounced.[1]

If most lower-class Puerto Ricans do not regard church opposition as a deterrent, they do raise other serious objections to birth control: it undermines male authority; it promotes infidelity; it is detrimental to health; it inhibits pleasure.

Male authority. Some men object to their wives' using contraceptives because they feel it robs them of rightful male authority.

[1] Robert C. Cook, *Human Fertility: The Modern Dilemma* (New York: William Sloane Associates, 1951), p. 338.

They hold that control in the sexual sphere belongs exclusively to the husband. This means that the husband may have extramarital sexual contacts, but can forbid these to his wife; and that he and not his wife will determine the time, form, and frequency of sexual relations. Birth control, then, is just one aspect of the sexual relationship which he feels is his domain.

I don't like to be governed by my wife. If she tries to use birth control I will leave her.

I am the one who avoids them (contraceptives). She doesn't know the secret of birth control. The woman gets pregnant if the man wants her to.

Fear of infidelity. Closely related to this point is the man's fear that allowing the wife to control conception will give her freedom to have sexual relations with other men. As mentioned previously, a man is extremely jealous and suspicious of his wife. At the same time, he tends to consider her naïve, lightheaded, and unable to reason as well as a man. He holds contrary views of men. Men are clever, wise, on the lookout for sexual relationships, and can easily win women over. Consequently, granting any freedom to the wife only makes it easier for some clever male to conquer her.

The husband assumes that fear of pregnancy is a deterrent to infidelity on the part of the wife. If she were to have a child while her husband was using birth control, he would then have positive proof that she was having an affair. If, on the other hand, the wife uses birth control, the husband cannot detect her illicit relations. A number of women in our sample expressed fear at suggesting female methods of birth control to their husbands:

If the woman is sterilized, the husband mistrusts her. He thinks the wife is unfaithful. You must keep all those things in mind.

I wanted to be sterilized but I didn't dare to tell him. Many men don't like their wives to be operated on because they think the women want this in order to have relations with other men.

This suspicion is a barrier to free communication between wives and husbands, a subject to be discussed later. It also leads to anxiety by women in whose families birth control is used, for if the method fails, there is always the danger that the husband will attribute pregnancy to illicit relations. Two clear examples of such anxiety are given below.

I heard of a woman here who used the diaphragm. Later she became pregnant, and the husband said the child was not his. They almost separated because, inasmuch as they were using birth control, the husband thought she was pregnant by another man.

(After I had nine children) I brought condoms home from the health center and he used them for about two years. Since I had my last child four months ago I haven't asked him to use them yet because I haven't menstruated. If he uses them and then finds out I am pregnant again, my husband might think I was having relations with other men; so I can't ask him to use them until I know whether I am pregnant or not.

Men may also, because of jealousy, forbid their wives to be examined by a male physician, thus keeping them from learning about contraception.

Health. The most frequently cited objection to the program is that it might impair one's health. Both men and women fear that birth control methods cause cancer and other dread diseases in women; that diaphragms get trapped in the vagina and require extraordinary measures to remove; and that sterilization may cause a woman to be chronically ill and "useless." While public health physicians in Puerto Rico are not subject to such misgivings, there is evidence that certain private physicians, either as a result of ignorance or religious fervor, do propagate such beliefs; and at least one religious organization is known to use such propaganda. In the absence of authoritative information to the contrary, it is not surprising that such beliefs are strong and tenacious.

73

I don't know any (birth control) methods. At the Public Health Unit they give instructions, but I fear them because people say it causes cancer.

I have never used prophylactics with my wife nor will I. That is dangerous because if it breaks the woman may die if that stays inside her womb.

Pleasure. The previous discussion has concentrated mainly on female contraceptives, suggesting that men preferred to control conception. While this is true, it does not mean that men have no objections to the condom. Nine out of every ten men in our sample objected to it, giving as their most frequent reason that it destroys the pleasure of the sexual act. It is true that rubber is a poor conductor of body warmth, and this may be what was meant. Other comments, however, suggest that for some, the diminished pleasure is a result of psychological as well as physical factors. To understand the psychological aspect it is necessary to know something about sexual relations in Puerto Rico.

As in other societies with a double standard of sexual morality, Puerto Rican men feel that there are two classes of women, "good" and "bad." Bad women are the prostitutes with whom one can really enjoy oneself sexually—but good women are the kind of girl whom one can marry. They are pure and good just as one's mother or sister and must be treated with courtesy, respect, and reserve. To some extent this attitude is maintained even in marriage. Sexual relations may become somewhat mechanical and nonerotic, both because the husband cannot get over the idea that his wife is a good and pure woman, and because his wife, brought up to regard sex as ugly and unladylike, may encourage this attitude by her own passivity or frigidity. For variety, or for a more sensual kind of sexual relationship, a man turns to the prostitute. To protect himself from venereal disease, he usually uses a contraceptive. He then comes to feel that the condom is part of the world of evil, and has no place in relationships with his wife. Using it at home would degrade a pure and sacred relationship.

74

Those things I don't use with my wife, because it debases my wife to use something that is used with prostitutes.

Those are used only with prostitutes, and my wife is an honest woman.

My husband says, "I am clean and my wife is clean, so we don't need to use those."

Perhaps it is for this reason that so many men speak of the condom as something dirty, and regard it as revolting and loathsome.

They are filthy . . . repulsive . . . I feel sick to my stomach.

I consider them filthy because of the disgust they give after one finishes the sexual act.

The complaint that the condom is less pleasurable thus appears to be based not only on purely physical factors, but also on other considerations that reduce the psychological pleasure of the sexual act.

Barriers to Communication of Birth Control Information

To be successful, a birth control program should provide for effective publicity and easily available information about aims and methods of birth control. In this matter Puerto Rico would appear to be in a favorable position. The birth control clinics have been in existence for over a decade; the newspapers have been full of arguments for and against birth control; and, as already indicated, the pulpit itself has inadvertently contributed to awareness of means for limiting births.

In nearly every family in our sample, both husbands and wives knew about sterilization, and in every family the husband knew about the condom. However, we discovered that frequently one spouse knew of methods which the other did not know. A similar pattern was discovered with respect to motivation. While both spouses might have had identical ideas about family size, one spouse frequently either did not know what the other spouse wanted, or assumed that more children were wanted than actually were. The explanation of these findings is that sexual matters are not a common topic of discussion between husband and wife. Women are brought up with great prudishness, are often ignorant of sex upon marriage, and are taught that modesty and reticence on sexual matters are important attributes of the good woman. At the same time, the male learns that it is not fitting to discuss such matters with a "good" woman—and by definition his wife is always a good woman. As stated earlier, a woman is very reluctant to suggest to her husband that she use contraceptive methods, lest he suspect her of wanting to engage in extramarital sexual activity without being detected. These are typical comments:

I have heard some of my friends talking about condoms, and I liked the idea. [Did you tell your husband?] No. I did not dare to. I never speak of those things with him. I get ashamed.

I don't know how he feels about that. I don't like to talk about certain things. I don't speak of those things with my husband. I feel ashamed.

To my wife? Me talk about these things? Look man, I couldn't even try. . . . I am not accustomed to talk about such things with my wife.

The wife would be offended if one used the condom. [Have you ever talked it over with her?] No, never. I would not dare to do it.

The decision to use birth control is usually a mutual one. Even if both partners have knowledge of birth control methods, little action can occur unless this knowledge is communicated by discussion. This is also true in the matter of motivation. If each partner thinks that the other wants a large family, little action will be taken. The couple will consider contraception only if both become aware that their wishes are identical.

Also important to know is which spouse is more influential in family decision-making. Where the man feels that it is his exclusive prerogative to initiate birth control, the wife's knowledge or attitudes may be irrelevant. A few men in the sample were surprised at the idea that women might have anything to say about this matter, and would consider it impertinent of them to suggest something that is obviously the man's business. When such a situation exists, it is a waste of effort to concentrate on the women in public health clinics. Since men are usually the least interested in birth control, appeals to them must be much more forceful if they are to be effective.

Modesty in women also impedes knowledge-seeking. Puerto Rican women are usually ashamed to ask for birth control information and materials. They are also ashamed to be examined by a male physician (many are ashamed at being seen by their own husbands), and some are even ashamed of being seen in a birth control clinic. Thus modesty is one of the major stumbling blocks to the program, for it obstructs both the seeking and sharing of information.

The preceding sections have described a number of cultural factors seriously hampering the effectiveness of the birth control program. Ambivalence about family size; fears that contraception will foster infidelity, undermine male authority, produce illness, or diminish pleasure; and barriers to communication of birth control information have all contributed to reluctance to use contraception. This does not mean, however, that birth control has been completely rejected. Of the seventy-two families studied by the Family Life Project, over two-thirds reported having some experience with contraception. Although many of these families discontinued birth control or use it ineffectively, we must account for their attempts.

It should be pointed out that cultural factors influence motivation not only where contraceptive methods are used but also where they are not practiced. One method that has proved increasingly attractive in Puerto Rico is sterilization. A review of the reasons will illustrate the interplay of culture, motivation, and the decision to accept or reject methods of controlling birth.

In 1950 close to one out of every five deliveries in Puerto Rican hospitals was followed by sterilization. Between four and five thousand sterilizations occur every year. This has not, however, produced any appreciable reduction in fertility as yet for several reasons; most deliveries do not occur in hospitals, the popularity of sterilization is relatively recent, and the operation is generally performed only after several pregnancies. But the demand for sterilizations continues to grow. Physicians turn down many women because of insufficient hospital bed space, or because they feel these particular women have not had enough children to merit the operation. Sterilization is so popular that local politicians dispense the necessary bed space in return for political allegiance. What explains this phenomenal popularity?

Sterilization is effective and relatively easy. As one woman put it, "It is only once, sure, and then you forget about it and don't have to use those dirty things." Another reason is that sterilization is usually performed in the hospital, postpartum, thus removing some of the onus and embarrassment of a special trip and a special examination. Yet by at least two criteria the measure is drastic. It requires an operation and it is irreversible; one cannot later change one's mind about wanting more children. Nevertheless, some families experiment with less drastic methods and switch later to sterilization; others try only this method. Our study showed that few people in the sample continued to use chemical or mechanical contraceptives, and either moved to sterilization, or stopped birth control altogether.

This trend away from birth "control" and toward sterilization can be explained by describing a pattern characteristic of many families whose case histories were collected.

In the early years of marriage little thought is given to fertility control. For various reasons, some of which we have indicated, the couple is eager to start a family, but reluctant to discuss matters pertaining to sex and childbearing. Consequently, when thought of family limitation occurs, it is usually the wife who feels concern. Too modest or fearful to seek information or discuss the matter with her husband, she cannot implement her desire to limit the size of her family, and no positive steps are taken. As a result, the Puerto Rican woman finds herself with as many children as she ever wants while she is still very young. By age twenty-five, for example, "more second births have occurred per 1,000 women on the island than occur in the United States by age 35."[2]

With three or four children, motivation for some kind of action becomes stronger. The family may begin to feel desperate and decide that something must be done that is swift and sure. The course of action chosen depends largely on the couple's knowledge of, and attitudes toward, birth control. If there is little knowledge or attitudes are strongly prejudicial, one or more children may be given away; the husband may desert the family; or sterilization, which is apparently known to everyone, will be sought. If knowledge and attitudes are different, ordinary birth control methods may be tried. At this point of high motivation, the availability of competent advice may be the deciding factor. Advice from a midwife, a public health nurse, or a physician is very likely to touch off action on birth control. Under such circumstances, the wife frequently breaks through the communication barrier, discusses the matter with her husband, gets his permission, and takes action.

By now, however, the couple is used to intercourse without mechanical devices and finds the prescribed techniques burdensome. Moreover, having conquered some of her modesty, the woman may discuss the matter with a married friend, who may tell her of the danger of contracting cancer. The husband may find the prescribed method tiresome, "unclean," or unpleasurable. Consequently, it is either discontinued or used erratically. Another pregnancy ensues. The family now feels that contraception is ineffective or impracticable and that something must be done once and for all. Sterilization provides an answer.

[2] J. W. Combs, Jr., and Kingsley Davis, "The Pattern of Puerto Rican Fertility," *Population Studies*, IV (March 1951), 371.

IMPLICATIONS

Possible Program Modifications

How can knowledge of the cultural influences at work in Puerto Rico help in planning a more effective birth control program? Such planning should take into account those cultural factors that bear most directly on public acceptance of the program, as well as take into account what is realistically possible. While new methods of contraception might minimize many of the current objections, much could be done to increase the effectiveness of existing facilities, in light of known cultural factors. It is of prime importance to improve methods of disseminating birth control information. If one were operating in a political vacuum, a public campaign with posters, leaflets, motion pictures, broadcasts, and mobile units might be the most effective method of spreading knowledge of contraception. However, the delicate nature of the subject makes it advisable to disseminate the information in quieter ways.

At the present time, the clinics are passive repositories of birth control materials. Even without a public campaign, greater efforts could be made to attract women to these clinics. These clinics are only one of about a dozen kinds of public health clinics. In all these others, physicians and nurses could influence their patients by stressing the bearing of excessive fertility on tuberculosis, malnutrition, and so on. The importance of the health and psychological well-being of *every child* could be stressed in children's clinics. Wherever possible, women could be referred to the prematernal birth control clinics.

Another aid to spreading knowledge of birth control practice would be premarital and marital counseling. Newlyweds could be apprised of the heavy responsibilities of parenthood *before* such status is achieved, thus stimulating early interest in birth control. If the public health agencies could not do this directly, they could at least encourage other agencies to do so. Moreover, since the communication block between husband and wife appears to be a crucial barrier to action, and since the Puerto Rican husband is the key figure in decision-making, every effort should be made to reach men. If husbands and wives are able to express themselves on sexual matters before a nurse or physician, a great step toward beneficial action would be taken. In revisits to some of the families in our sample, interviewers found that several women had begun to practice birth control merely because they had talked about it. As one woman put it, "I'd always been ashamed before. But after talking with you, I was able to talk to my husband about it." The interviewers did no propagandizing. Bringing the subject out into the open had furnished enough impetus to bring about action.

Measures to reduce embarrassment in the clinic would also aid in spreading birth control practice. Utilizing more nurses and female physicians, exercising greater tact, and conducting pelvic examinations only when absolutely necessary, would eliminate a great deal of embarrassment for patients.

Once in the clinic, it is not enough to present the patient with materials and to give instruction on their use. Ill-founded fears concerning birth control must be dispelled, some hints provided as to what to tell the husband, and the importance of continuing control measures stressed. Puerto Rican lower-class women are too modest and too respectful of authority to ask many questions. Their inner questions must be anticipated and dealt with by discussion or lecture methods. Toward the same end efforts could be made to set up discussion groups for mothers, to facilitate the open consideration of problems and tabooed topics.

Finally, it is important that public health personnel themselves have adequate knowledge of the culture of the particular group with which they are dealing. Members of a higher-class group often demonstrate considerable ignorance about lower-class groups in their own society. Discussions with social workers and social scientists working with such groups can teach these people a great deal about their own culture. Moreover, workers should realize the great importance of working simultaneously toward the reduction of fertility and mortality in areas of population pressure. To many public health personnel, the prematernal clinic is just one of many clinics and one whose importance their own training and dispositions may lead them to minimize.

6

Interpersonal Influence in
Family Planning in Puerto Rico*

In areas of the world where illiteracy is high and levels of living are low, the mass media play a relatively minor role in determining the opinions and knowledge of large numbers of the population. In such regions, word-of-mouth communications via primary groups or local opinion leaders are of greater importance. The introduction of technological change in such areas can be facilitated by the identification of the important influence groups or persons, and by knowledge of the processes by which these shape and communicate information and opinion. In this chapter three topics will be discussed: (1) the *extent* of interpersonal communication on birth control; (2) the *sources* of influence and information; (3) the possible differential effects of these sources on fertility control behavior among a sample of lower-income Puerto Ricans.

THE EXTENT OF INTERPERSONAL
COMMUNICATION ON BIRTH CONTROL

The sample under consideration is composed of 888 women and a subsample of 322 husbands of these women. All families had at least one child, had less than eight years of education (2.7

* This chapter written in collaboration with Kurt Back and Reuben Hill.

and 4.0 median years education for females and males), and were chosen from general out-patient clinics and birth control clinics throughout the island in such a fashion as to include a roughly equal number of sterilized cases, and of current, past, and never users of birth control.

Chapter 5 has referred to the blocks to communication on sexual matters which exist between husband and wife in the lower-class Puerto Rican family. In view of this, it is of some significance that as many as 44 percent of the males and 56 percent of the females replied affirmatively to the question, "Do you ever talk with your friends about birth control?"—indicating for both sexes considerable discussion of this topic outside the conjugal unit. The higher proportion of wives who discuss this topic with friends probably reflects their greater motivation. (That the difference is not due to a greater tendency on the part of the women to discuss *everything* with friends is shown by the fact that men score higher than women on discussion with friends of religion and future plans. Wives, moreover, are found to be substantially better informed than their husbands on sources of supply of birth control materials, perhaps showing the effect of greater pooling of information.)

Moving to questions of greater specificity, we may inquire as to the extent of interpersonal influence as regards *particular decisions* concerning family limitation. In this connection the distribution of responses to four questions is relevant:

(1) When you first thought your family was large enough, was there anyone with whom you talked who made you think you had enough children? (Asked of those who have the same as or more than their ideal number of children.)

(2) When you first started using birth control, was there anyone with whom you talked who made you think about using birth control? (Asked of ever-users of birth control.)

(3) How did you find out about the first method you used?

(4) How did you find out about the second method you used?

Table 4 tells us the extent to which members of the sample

disclaim the influence of "outside" sources; that is, they claim the motivation or the knowledge came only from themselves.

Table 4. Members of sample citing no sources other than self

	Males		Females	
Question number	(%)	Number	(%)	Number
(1)	63.0	(247)	43.7	(732)
(2)	66.6	(258)	34.0	(676)
(3)	16.0	(244)	0.0	(675)
(4)	15.2	(144)	0.0	(437)

We note again the importance of interpersonal influence, and again that the wives appear to be much more exposed to it than husbands. However, at least two alternative explanations are possible for the latter finding. First, the authoritarian male, characteristic of this class of Puerto Rican society, may like to think, or to have the interviewer think, that he makes up his own mind. As a special instance of this, since the questions do not exclude spouse as source, husbands may be reluctant to admit being informed or motivated by their wives. Second, with regard to methods of birth control, males learn about techniques much earlier than females, and consequently may be more likely to forget the source. Moreover, they may be reluctant to attribute the source of knowledge to prostitutes, or, again, to their wives.

THE SOURCE OF INTERPERSONAL INFLUENCE

Among those in the sample who do cite others as affecting their knowledge and attitudes, what persons or categories of persons stand out as influential? Let us first present the unweighted average of the first three questions above to get an overall picture (Table 5).

Table 5. Source of influence and information, by sex
(unweighted average of questions 1–3, in percent)

Sources	Male	Female
Friends and Neighbors	39.9	27.9
Clinic Personnel	10.6	20.7
Spouse	9.4	17.9
Kin	17.4	15.1
Mother, mother-in-law	8.9	13.9
Other (Social worker, mid- wife, unspecified)	13.8	4.5
Total	100.0	100.0

We are struck first by the relative infrequency with which spouses cite each other as sources of influence or information. It is possible that some of the individuals were taking their spouses' influence for granted and did not mention it; yet the consistency of this datum with previous evidence of lack of communication on these topics might suggest validity.

A second point of interest is the large representation of mothers or mothers-in-law, a group which stands on a par with spouses as a source of orientation for both sexes. The hypothesis that mother-child bonds in Puerto Rico may be stronger than the husband-wife has been explored elsewhere; yet the strong taboos on discussion in this area of sex and reproduction make this datum initially surprising.

In the light of strong kinship ties, we might have expected kin to figure more prominently than friends and neighbors, though intrafamilial taboos on sex discussion is consistent with this finding.

Differences between the sexes are according to expectation. With more rigidly circumscribed social worlds, women more frequently cite close relatives (husbands and mothers) while males, with a wider range of social contacts, more frequently cite friends, neighbors, and "others."

86

Finally, clinic sources, while important, are perhaps less frequently mentioned than might have been expected from a sample weighted with women exposed to such clinics (47 percent of the women have at some time obtained birth control materials from the clinics). It might be argued, however, that the table mainly reflects historical influences and does not imply current reference figures or groups. Thus, for example, it might be supposed that the clinics *now* stand out in women's minds as prime sources for advice and information, though they may not have happened to be prime movers in the past. In this connection, a question asked of female respondents is quite revealing: "If you were to consult with someone other than your husband about the proper number of children to have, with whom would it be?" Only 16 percent mentioned nurses, physicians, or the clinics. A third cited friends and relatives, somewhat over a third relatives, 10 percent mothers and about 3 percent "others." Thus the current reference groups very much resemble those important in the past, and the clinic as a source of counsel remains of relatively minor importance.

While Table 5 has provided an overall picture, we now need to turn to the specific questions which formed the basis for the average figures cited in this table. Table 6 includes the fourth question as well.

It seems reasonable to assume that the questions (at least 1 through 3) run from less intimate to more intimate, from general advice on ends to specific information on means. It is interesting that the *direction* of the percentages runs similarly for both sexes —friends-neighbors, spouse, and clinic sources tending to increase as specificity rises, while all other categories tend to decline. This similarity could be partially explained if both spouses received advice from the same source. In view of the strong taboos on cross-sex discussions, this seems unlikely, though one member of the pair might report a source which was in contact with him indirectly *through* his or her spouse. Certainly the upward trend in clinic source for males would support the latter hypothesis, since the prematernal clinics are for females.

Table 6. Sources of influence and information for those who cited
source, by sex (in percent)

Sources	(1) Who made you think you had enough children?	(2) Who made you think about using birth control?	(3) Where found out about first method used?	(4) Where found out about second method used?
Females				
Friends-neighbors	23.1	29.3	31.1	26.0
Clinic-profess.	11.8	23.0	27.4	35.2
Spouse	10.0	16.4	27.5	27.3
Kin	23.2	16.9	7.6	7.4
Mother–mother-in-law	29.2	9.7	2.8	0.7
Other	2.7	4.7	3.6	3.4
Total	100.0	100.0	100.0	100.0
Number of cases	(412)	(423)	(651)	(420)
Males				
Friends-neighbors	22.9	41.7	55.0	39.4
Clinic-profess.	5.4	8.3	18.0	33.6
Spouse	6.5	11.5	10.3	14.0
Kin	32.6	16.3	3.4	5.7
Mother–mother-in-law	19.6	7.0	—	—
Other	13.0	15.2	13.3	7.3
Total	100.0	100.0	100.0	100.0
Number of cases	(92)	(86)	(205)	(122)

It is also possible that the same forces are operating with both
sexes; that is, that as intimacy and specification of advice rise,
influence groups will tend toward the two extremes of intimacy

—the most intimate (husband and wife) and the least intimate (clinic and neighbor-friends). The decline in kin and mother influence may be due to the taboos on sex discussion among family members, taboos which do not apply so strongly to friends and clinic staff on the one hand, or to husbands and wives on the other. Thus the mother and other kin give *general* advice, less intimate individuals (other than spouses), specific advice. It is now clear that the prominence of mothers noted in the average figures in Table 5 is attributable mainly to the first question, and almost exclusively to the first and second questions.

In discussing the paucity of spouse references in Table 5, we suggested the possibility that such sources are taken for granted and thus not mentioned. However, this would probably not apply to wives' first source of information on birth control, yet we see that only 27 percent of the wives learned about the first methods used from their husbands. This is especially low when we consider that 70 percent of the women learned about their first method *after* marriage.

One point worthy of brief comment is the fact that most of the friends and neighbors who give advice are older rather than the same age as or younger than the recipient of advice. In the case of females the unweighted mean percentage of advising friends or neighbors older than the respondent is 84 ranging from 80 to 86 percent over the four items; in the case of males the mean percentage is 64, ranging from 52 to 72 percent.

More needs to be said of the "kin" category, which thus far has only been noted generally. If our hypothesis according to intimacy is true, we would expect that the *closer* kin relationships would be more frequently represented in the areas of greater intimacy.

If we consider the close relationships to be those of the nuclear family (brother, sister, and father), it is apparent that the hypothesis is borne out. All three categories decline sharply, while other relationships remain the same or rise, though erratically.

Table 7. Breakdown of "kin" category into specific relationships, female only (in percent)

Relationship	Questions			
	(1)	(2)	(3)	(4)
Sister[a]	37.4	30.6	20.9	28.6
Sister-in-law	7.3	22.7	29.1	22.8
Comadre[b]	13.6	20.0	10.4	20.0
Aunt	13.6	13.3	12.5	11.4
Father or father-in-law	12.5	2.7	—	—
Brother or brother-in-law	5.2	—	—	—
Female cousin	2.1	2.7	16.7	17.2
Other (niece, godmother, grandparent, unspecified)	8.3	8.0	10.4	
Total	100.0	100.0	100.0	100.0
Number of cases	(96)	(75)	(48)	(35)

[a] Practically all cases in this category are older sisters.
[b] Woman who serves as godmother for one's child.

Male kin are conspicuous by their absence, present to any extent only in the first and least intimate category, reflecting, of course, cross-sex discussion.

DIFFERENTIAL EFFECTS

What differential effect, if any, does the source of motivation or knowledge have on its recipients? One way of looking at this would be to classify recipients according to the predominant direction of their sources of attitude and knowledge. Let us take the 690 women who have ever used a birth control method and type them according to their predominant source of orientation. We shall define "predominant source" as that class of reference individuals mentioned in at least two of the first three questions. If different sources are named for all three questions, the predominant source of orientation will be classified as "multi-

Table 8. Predominant source of orientation for attitude and knowledge with respect to family planning (in percent)

Self	17.9
Husband	13.1
Kin	14.9
Neighbor-friend	17.1
Clinic	11.9
Multi-group	25.1
Total	100.0
Number of cases	(690)

group." Table 8 shows the distribution of types by this system of classification.

When these groups are examined with respect to their demographic makeup (residence, marital type, education, age, and age at marriage) with few exceptions the types seem to be randomly distributed. However, the self-oriented are much more urban and the neighbor-friend much more rural than other groups; and the clinic-oriented are somewhat older than the sample as a whole.

Our first question will be to determine whether or not these types are associated with knowledge of and time of initiation of

Table 9. Knowledge and initiation of birth control, by orientation types (in percent)

	Median Birth after which first method was learned	Median number of methods known	Median birth after which first method was started
Self	1.42	6.33	3.30
Husband	1.26	6.83	3.20
Kin	0.37	6.84	3.30
Neighbor-friend	1.70	6.92	3.30
Clinic	2.08	6.48	3.60
Multi-group	1.22	6.57	2.90
Mean for sample	1.39	6.64	3.10

birth control. We are struck, first of all, by the relatively poor showing of the clinic-oriented. They are the latest to learn, know fewer methods than all but one group, and start birth control somewhat later than the sample as a whole. We might speculate that these are individuals who have been relatively isolated from the more typical influence of friends and kin which might be expected to operate early within a marriage. In the absence of such informal pressures, motivations for birth control use may develop more slowly, as a result of growing economic pressures. When pressure becomes strong, these individuals seek professional guidance either because they lack primary group sources toward which to turn, or because they feel it too late to rely on nonprofessional advice. In the light of the hypothesis of economic pressure, it is interesting that 45 percent of this group cited economic reasons for starting birth control, as compared with an average of 35 percent for the entire sample. Moreover, that this group leans toward the clinic as its reference group is seen by the fact that 25 percent state that they would prefer to go to a doctor or nurse if they wanted advice on family planning, where only 20 percent of the total sample would so prefer.

The self-oriented, however, are equally free from primary group influence, yet have learned more and started birth control earlier than the clinic-oriented. This group is strongly urban and somewhat better educated than the general sample. Possibly the self-oriented are more highly motivated early in marriage, not waiting for fertility to take its course as do the families who later become clinic-oriented.

Finally, kin-oriented are early learners of birth control, but multi-group oriented emerge both as early learners and earliest starters. Let us see if any patterns emerge as we examine, in turn, type of methods used (Table 10), and regularity and effectiveness of them (Table 11).

Two groups stand out in one way or another—the clinic-oriented and the husband-oriented. How they stand out can best be illustrated by extracting certain categories and combinations

Table 10. Pattern of birth control use among ever-users, by predominant influence types (in percent)

Type	Self	Husband	Kin	Neighborfriend	Clinic	Multigroup	Mean
Natural methods only	15.7	22.8	13.5	10.3	3.7	14.4	13.6
Sterilization only	11.6	5.4	10.6	10.3	12.3	15.5	11.5
Mechanical-chemical only	19.8	14.1	27.9	29.1	43.2	23.6	25.5
Mechanical-chemical and natural	31.4	34.8	30.8	30.8	22.2	31.0	30.5
Sterilization and other	21.5	22.9	17.3	19.5	18.6	15.5	18.9
Total	100.0	100.0	100.1	100.0	100.0	100.0	100.0
Number of cases	(121)	(92)	(104)	(117)	(81)	(174)	(689)

of categories from Table 10 and expressing these in summary fashion:

	Clinic		Husband		Total sample
	%	Rank	%	Rank	%
Ever used natural methods	25.9	(Lowest)	57.6	(Highest)	44.1
Used mechan.-chem. only	43.2	(Highest)	14.1	(Lowest)	25.5
Used combinations of types	40.8	(Lowest)	57.7	(Highest)	49.4

Those whose predominant orientation are their husbands are most likely to have used natural methods (largely withdrawal), least likely to have used mechanical-chemical methods exclusively, and most likely to have used different classes of methods. The reverse is true for the clinic-oriented. Thus we might say that whereas the clinic-oriented tend to use exclusively the means provided by the clinic, the husband-oriented are *experimentalists*, trying out different methods but leaning toward those which

(1) may be best known to the husband; (2) may require a maximum of cooperation. With regard to the first point it is significant that 65 percent of those women who learned about their first method from their husbands were told about a *natural* method, whereas only 25 percent of the entire sample learned a natural technique as their first method. With regard to the latter point, we should note that interspousal communication scores both on general topics and on topics specific to birth control are higher for the husband-oriented group than for any other.

We now move to a consideration of the persistence and effectiveness with which birth control is used by the various groups.

Table 11. Persistence and success of birth control, by predominant influence types (in percent)

Type	Short-term irregular use	Long-term regular use	Failure rate[a] (median)
Self	35.5	14.9	0.047
Husband	31.5	32.6	0.042
Kin	40.4	12.5	0.052
Neighbor-friend	34.1	18.8	0.052
Clinic	25.6	28.0	0.038
Multi-group	36.2	20.2	0.048
Mean for sample	34.5	20.4	0.048

[a] Unplanned pregnancies since birth control was started per month of exposure to conception from that time to time of interview or time of sterilization.

Again the clinic- and husband-oriented groups stand out, but this time at the same rather than opposite poles. Both groups are lowest in short-term irregular use, highest in long-term regular use, and lowest in failure rates. We are not surprised that the clinic group should be outstanding in this regard, but why should the husband-oriented group, which displayed the highest proportion of natural users and experimenters (which might be interpreted as erratic users), be equally persistent and effective?

Although this is a difficult question to answer in any definite fashion, we may suggest the following explanation.

The husband-oriented group is successful precisely because effective birth control use is enhanced by the cooperation of husband and wife. Even though the methods used are intrinsically less effective, this deficiency can to a large degree be counterbalanced by *joint responsibility* in the execution of family limitation. The fact that women in this group received their predominant motivation for birth control use from their husbands (assuming that the women themselves were interested) suggests that such joint responsibility was present—and that *despite* the use of relatively inefficient methods and a high degree of experimentation, persistent and effective utilization of birth control ensued. Indeed, experimentation itself may express not erratic or random behavior, but a search for more workable methods of family limitation.

With regard to the clinic-oriented, we may suggest a corresponding hypothesis. High persistence and success among this group is achieved without the same degree of husband orientation because of (1) the intrinsic efficiency of the methods employed, and (2) because of the relatively "late start" which may have induced anxiety for success.

A general conclusion which follows from these hypotheses is that a combination of clinical methods and husband orientation (i.e., joint responsibility) would provide a more effective pattern of birth control use than is evidenced by any of the groups in the sample.

CONCLUSIONS

We have seen that there is a not inconsiderable amount of discussion between members of the sample and others on the subject of birth control. Such discussion appears to affect positively its recipients' motivation on starting family planning, as well as their knowledge of specific birth control methods, although this influence tends to be felt or admitted more often by females than by males. On the whole, friends and neighbors appear to be the most frequent sources of influence, especially for males, and mothers are mentioned with considerable frequency. Citation of spouse as a source is surprisingly infrequent, and the clinics, while important, are not mentioned as frequently as might have been expected in the present sample.

In a single area of behavior, fertility control, we have seen the differential contributions of various influence groups or individuals. As initial *motivators* toward fertility control, close relatives other than spouse seem of major importance. *Prescribers*, however, are infrequently drawn from such sources and tend toward less intimate figures such as clinic personnel and friends, or toward the most intimate relative—the spouse.

As an ideal type construction, we see the lower-class Puerto Rican wife early in marriage as unconcerned about fertility control and/or reluctant to discuss such matters with her husband. After a number of children, however, she seeks out or is sought out by close relatives who pressure her to "do something." She then turns to other sources for specific advice on what to do. Indeed, perhaps partly as a result of such pressures, she overcomes her earlier reluctance and discusses such matters with her husband.

We noted that in that minority of cases where the wife's principal reference individual was the husband, length and regularity of birth control practice was especially marked, and failure of methods lower than average despite the utilization of intrinsically inefficient methods. This supports the commonsense notion that the success of a cooperative venture is facilitated by agreement and communication on means and ends. That spouses in Puerto Rico more typically turn to extraconjugal sources for motivation and prescription on birth control is another evidence of the cultural blocks in family organization which impede the realization of small family goals. It has been shown that this shortcoming may to some extent be compensated for by a "clinic-orientation" on the part of the wife, an orientation which implies the use of intrinsically effective methods. However, for a number of reasons, those clinics are not used to any great extent by the general population, and, as shown above, tend to be used relatively late in childbearing.

7

The Bishops, Politics,
and Birth Control

On October 1, 1960, at 5 A.M., the usually tranquil village of Barranquitas, Puerto Rico, was awakened by vociferous chanting from a nearby hill. "Viva Cristo Rey! Viva the Pope! Viva the Most Holy Virgin!" The crowd, huddled against the dark and the early morning chill, was facing a small altar on which a statue of the Virgin stood out against a background of broad-leafed tropical foliage. Soon the melancholy rhythm of a thousand toneless voices reciting the Rosary could be heard. What had motivated so many Puerto Ricans, usually apathetic toward their religion, to leave their homes before dawn for public prayer? The mystery was soon dispelled, for a public address system sent the following message ringing from the hilltop: "The objective of the party is to bring Christ to government so that His will be done on earth as it is in heaven. His will should be done in government, in the Senate, in the House, in business, in industry, and in labor. . . . Our social program is based on Catholic social doctrine as expressed by the Popes." What had appeared to be a prayer meeting was in fact a political rally for the newly formed Christian Action Party (PAC)—a party whose official insignia was the rosary, whose meeting places were often the churches, and whose inspiration sprung from the Roman Catholic creed and clergy.

The emergence of the PAC was astonishing to most Puerto Ricans, for the island brand of Catholicism is generally nominal.

But if they were astonished at PAC, they were overwhelmed when the Bishops issued a pastoral letter labeling it a sin to vote for the party in power, the Popular Democratic Party. The shock was evident in the editorials of the leading newspapers. *El Mundo* headlined its editorial "A Tragedy" and the *San Juan Star* announced that "the Bishops have sinned against the people . . . against their country . . . and against the Church." *El Imparcial* maintained that "the Puerto Rican Catholic hierarchy has cracked the foundations of the traditions and veneration of 468 years of its Church."

Apparently counting on the relatively mild Catholicism of most Puerto Ricans and their strong tradition of separation of Church and State, Popular leaders grasped the Bishops' statement almost gleefully and turned it into their main campaign issue. The mayor of one of the largest towns reported that attendance at Popular party meetings more than doubled following the Bishops' letter, while another leader held that "what the party needs is three more bishops." Thundering that it represented "the gravest danger to liberty to the island since Christopher Columbus discovered Puerto Rico," Governor Muñoz Marín barnstormed the villages and rural districts, exhorting Puerto Ricans to maintain their liberty by voting the Popular ticket.

The result was the bitterest and most emotional campaign ever witnessed in Puerto Rico, and acts in defiance of the clergy abounded. One senator called for an investigation of the Bishops for violation of the Puerto Rican constitution. Church walkouts and picketing and boycotting of churches were not infrequent. *Vivas* for the Pope were returned in some places by the chant "Mass yes, politics no"; and in San Juan hundreds of students and professionals carried black flags in a lengthy "March of Silence."

Some fervid Catholics became vitriolic. In a letter criticizing the anti-Bishop stand of the *Island Times*, a doctor wrote, "You can be honored by kissing the soil where [the Bishops] set their feet . . . you idiots and liars . . . your bitter and dirty tongues."

Priests, monseigneurs, and bishops joined with Catholic lay leaders in denouncing the government leaders as "neo-pagan," "atheist," "anti-Christian," and "heretical." Political leaflets linked the government in power with divorce, illegitimacy, crime, delinquency, pornography, abortion, and fiendish experiments on humans. The militant Catholic Youth Organization staged a huge book burning in the central plaza of Cayey, and their official newspaper, *Juventud*, proudly editorialized, *"We are ready to burn every Protestant Bible in Puerto Rico."*

Other devout Catholics who were also loyal Populars were torn by powerful conflicting emotions. "Tears flooded my eyes," wrote one such person to a newspaper, "as I read a pastoral letter issued last Sunday by their Excellencies the Archbishop and Bishops of Puerto Rico. For a Catholic, convinced of the truth in our divine Revelation, and for a Puerto Rican, proud of our island's freedom and social progress, that letter was an unexpected storm, stirring terrible conflicts in a worried heart." The issue caused acrimonious and painful conflicts not only within the individual conscience, but within institutions (e.g., the Bar Association voted 417 to 188 against the Bishops after protracted and heated debate) and even within families. As an extreme example of the latter, on the very day that Monseigneur Nazario, Chancellor of the Ponce Diocese, announced that "he who publicly approves of the program of the Popular Party with its heretical content not only commits a grave mortal sin but can also be excommunicated," the sister of one of the Bishops joined the Bishop's cousin in publicly announcing that she would vote Popular and not obey this "imposition." (She subsequently retracted her statement.)

What lay behind the Bishops' choice of a stand almost preordained to defeat, a stand censured by Catholic prelates in areas as disparate as Boston and Mexico? At least one thing seems certain. The decision was a hasty one accompanied by relatively little planning. It is true that politics are not new to Ponce's Bishop McManus, the island's leading exponent of the Church

Militant. According to an *Imparcial* columnist writing in 1953, the then Rector of the Catholic University of Ponce denounced McManus to the Vatican for meddling in Puerto Rican politics, for violent attacks on the governor, and for publication of a newspaper (*Luz y Verdad*) for the purpose of making political propaganda. On the other hand, the timing of the emergence of the PAC and the timing and pattern of subsequent clerical announcements all suggest a last-minute decision.

The party itself sprung up suddenly only a few months before the elections, the precipitating event being the House's tabling of a bill for released time for religious education. An almost blasé rejection of the bill and the intransigence of the government leaders in the face of Church demands caused considerable irritation in Catholic circles, while a great deal of confidence was inspired by the huge crowds which demonstrated in favor of the bill. A rather frantic scramble to get the required number of signatures to register the party ensued. In Bishop McManus' words, however, "the cup was filled to overflowing" when the Popular Party published its official program. In an apparent reference to legislation on divorce and birth control, the party stated that it could only prohibit acts which were immoral according to the general consensus of the Puerto Rican people, and that to prohibit acts which a respectable part of the population regarded as not immoral would be illicit in a regime of liberty. To the Bishops this was a clear case of "moral relativism," and, only weeks before the election, they released their pastoral letters.

From this point on no hypothesis other than lack of planning seems to account for the incredible series of Church announcements and "clarifications," each one of which seemed further to confuse Catholics and further to delight the Populars. Most of these centered around the question of whether the failure to follow the Bishops' demand on voting would constitute a sin. When San Juan's Bishop Davis was asked point blank on October 21, he replied, "There are no penalties involved; it is a matter between a Catholic and his conscience." On October 23, Cardinal Spellman was quoted in Puerto Rico as saying that disobedience would involve no penalty and consequently could not be considered a sin. Two days later McManus questioned the news story on Spellman, and maintained that disobedience was indeed a sin, whether or not a penalty was attached. On October 27 he stated that "there is no such thing as a sin without punishment," and on the following day the Chancellor of the Ponce Diocese wrote a letter to *El Mundo* in order to "avoid confusions" and to "make clear the moral position which Catholics have to assume." In this letter he stated that "every Catholic commits a grave sin if he votes for the Popular Party" and that a "grave mortal sin" and danger of excommunication is incurred for publicly supporting the Popular Party. Hardly had this clarification been issued when McManus announced that Chancellor Nazario had only been voicing a personal point of view. "In theory, however, it is not erroneous," he added cryptically. When Cardinal Spellman further confused the issue by lunching with Governor Muñoz without apology and with no apparent signs of contamination, McManus explained that the Cardinal had been tricked and given a "Judas' kiss" by the Governor. On November 4 an unnamed spokesman for Archbishop Davis stated that the Puerto Rican hierarchy was not happy with Spellman's statements nor with those of other high Church officials of the United States. He made it clear that the Puerto Rican bishops are responsible to the Vatican alone. He also stated that "naturally" those who vote Popular commit a sin, but added a most provocative sentence: "However, as the vote is secret, the priests will have no way of establishing how Catholics voted, unless they decide to reveal this vote in the confessional."

The bewildering series of communiques led one Puerto Rican to complain in a letter to the *San Juan Star:* "As a Catholic, I can vote without sinning since I reside in the diocese of San Juan. Had I been a resident of the Southern diocese I would presumably commit a sin." On November 7, however, the Archbishop of San Juan made the last announcement before the election, and took away any remaining vestiges of comfort for residents of San Juan. Ignoring the questions of penalties and of venial versus mortal sin, the Archbishop stated simply, "It is a sin for a Catholic to give his vote to the Popular Democratic Party."

Just before making this statement, Bishop Davis had been visiting the mainland, and when called upon to justify the pastoral letters, made a statement which local politicians had to read several times before believing their eyes: "If Puerto Rico had achieved democracy to the extent of the United States . . . it would not be necessary to issue such a letter. But in Puerto Rico . . . the pastoral had to be issued because of the ignorance of the people on political and religious matters." Full-page ads featuring this quotation immediately appeared in the major newspapers with the caption, "This is what the Bishop thinks of the Puerto Rican people."

The eve of the election found Muñoz confident and defiant, the Church leaders for the first time in a conciliatory mood. Muñoz had made a radio broadcast on November 4 "clarifying" the Popular position by supporting God, Christian morality, and the Ten Commandments. On these slim grounds Bishop Davis announced on November 6 that the Church "is open to conciliation" and that if Muñoz's message was received officially, they would give it "the most serious consideration." Perhaps not wanting to give up a good thing, Muñoz spurned the olive branch, retorting, "It is up to the voters."

After the voters gave Muñoz 58 percent of their votes and PAC only 6 percent, the question of sin burned more brightly than ever. Despite apparent pre-election agreement on the absence of any ecclesiastical penalty, leading Populars and their wives were refused communion on the Sunday following the election in at least five communities reported in the press. "Very pious women" were reported to have left the churches weeping after the refusals. In one community a family charged that their father, a leading Popular, had been denied a funeral service by the local priest.

On November 20 a circular letter issued by the Archdiocese of San Juan was read at Mass throughout the island. It took the stiffest line yet announced, exceeding in zealousness even the earlier pronouncements from the Ponce diocese. It held that anyone who makes a public statement that he does not repent his sin cannot receive the sacraments until he has "publicly withdrawn from the state of sin and made public atonement for his (or her) scandal or bad conduct." The letter provided needed support for the pastor of the San Juan cathedral, Reverend Tomas Maisonet, who had gained international fame by announcing he would deny communion to one of the Western Hemisphere's most popular women—San Juan mayoress Felisa Rincón. After the circular letter, Reverend Maisonet said that the mayoress would be expected to recant publicly "through radio, television or newspapers" before she could receive communion. He maintained that all Catholics who voted for the Popular Party committed a "mortal sin" and concluded, with unswerving logic, that "Puerto Rico today is a country of people in sin." Doña Felisa vociferously denied she had sinned, refused to repent, and, a devout Catholic, prayed for the misguided priest.

On November 22 her prayers were answered. From Chicago, Archbishop McManus declared that such statements had not been authorized by him, that the Church would not punish those who had disobeyed the order, that sacraments would not be denied anyone, and that his words applied to the three dioceses.

What had the Bishops and the PAC really wanted? Mayoress Felisa Rincón claimed they wanted a Catholic republic, and at times the party spokesmen indeed seemed to want a kingdom of God on earth. PAC candidate for governor, Salvador Perea Roselló, recommended that the insular constitution be amended to read, "God is the source of public power," rather than "the will of the people." The candidate for resident commissioner in Washington, Jorge Luis Córdova Díaz, in condemning Puerto

Rico's "atheist schools," stated that "nothing on earth is important except as a preparation for the eternal life," and Representative José Feliú Pesquera demanded that Christ be brought "to
the House, to the Senate, to all homes, to all professions." But if
these were PAC's general goals, its specific objectives boiled
down to two—religious education and abrogation of permissive
laws on birth control.

Of the two, the latter was the clearer issue, received the greater
share of attention, and had the longer history as an issue in Puerto
Rico. As Eduardo Flores, secretary of PAC, put it, "If it is a sin
to practice birth control, then it is a grave matter of conscience
to vote for a political party that sustains birth control laws . . .
the appeal of the new party is based almost exclusively on PAC
support of religious instruction for public schools and its objection to existing legislation on birth control and abortion." When
a Vatican spokesman was asked to comment on the Bishops'
pastorals, he justified them on only two grounds—that the
Bishops were within their authority, and that "for a number of
years the Puerto Rican religious and moral situation has been one
of particular gravity . . . it is sufficient to recall the intensive
campaign which occurred there in favor of birth control." One
of the few concrete planks in the PAC platform was the formation of a "Department of the Family" within the insular government "for the protection and exaltation of the Family." Among
those qualities of the family in line for protection and exaltation
were not only "prosperity" and "stability" but *fecundity*." In
its published program, the party promised to abrogate (*derogar*)
all legislation which "converts marriage into a mere instrument
of animal pleasure, which permits and develops free love, con-
cubinage, adultery, prostitution, abortion, neomalthusianism and
sterilization."

"Neomalthusianism," typically sandwiched between adultery
and prostitution, was the term used by Catholics to identify the
advocacy of birth control, and the particular target of the campaign became the rescinding of insular laws passed in 1936 per-

mitting the dissemination of contraceptive advice and materials in public clinics. While this might seem an attractive issue for a population roughly 80 percent Catholic, it might also seem anomalous that the issue needed to be raised at all. How could such laws be passed, and what has the reaction of the Catholic population been to them for the past two decades? The answers to these questions yield an interesting piece of social history, and provide some clues as to what may be expected in other Catholic countries as birth control information becomes widespread.

The religious monopoly of the Church ceased in 1898 with the annexation of Puerto Rico by the United States. Protestant missionaries and government officials soon arrived in considerable numbers, and while no striking inroads in the way of religious conversions were made immediately, the clear separation of Church and State, and the Protestantism of the top leadership paved the way for reforms of a non-Catholic nature. Private birth control organizations were established as early as 1926, and again, along with a clinic, in 1932. In both instances the ventures were short-lived as a result of Catholic action.

Significant developments in this field did not begin until the New Deal administration in Washington helped the emergence of a young and liberal local leadership in Puerto Rico. In 1935, fifty-three clinics were established under the auspices of a federal agency, but heavy pressure in Washington, reputedly from American Catholic sources, caused federal support to be withdrawn within a year. A number of clinics were reopened under private sponsorship, funded by continental and insular philanthropists. On May 15, 1937, the now famous Law 136 legalizing the teaching and practice of birth control was passed. In the temporary absence of Governor Winship, it was signed by Acting Governor Menéndez Ramos, but it is important to note that the law was passed by the elected legislature and strongly supported by the Acting Governor. On the strength of the law and a subsequent decision in the U.S. district court, the Insular Department of Health set up a system of prematernal clinics which provided for advice and free contraceptive materials in the 160 public health units and subunits of the island. The system represents one of the most extensive systems of public family planning facilities in the world. Although the Acting Governor was excommunicated, and the Church made formal protests, reaction to the law seemed both unorganized and *pro forma*. This absence of intensive opposition continued throughout the 1940's, and there were rumors of a gentleman's agreement between the Church and government to the effect that if the clinics were not aggressive about their program or about case finding, the Church would not be aggressive either. For whatever reason, the Department of Health never made serious efforts to inform the public about the contraceptive facilities, and the case loads of the clinics were modest in terms of the facilities and the need. Yearly new admissions ranged between four and five thousand, with a total active case load of only about fifteen thousand in 1950.

If there was ever any understanding between government and the hierarchy, it began to fade in the 1950's, and Church opposition stepped up markedly. Undoubtedly this was related to the appointment of the zealous James McManus as Bishop of Ponce in the late 1940's. Of equal plausibility as an explanation was the growing evidence that new organizational and scientific developments were making birth control a much greater threat to the Church than ever before.

The first evidence must have come from the extraordinary popularity of female sterilization, a method so widespread that women began to refer to it as simply "the operation." Surveys disclosed that the average lower-class Puerto Rican favored a family size of two or three children and approved the idea of family planning. Educational experiments with populations in small villages disclosed that Puerto Ricans were responsive to information and appeals about birth control. That the results of such studies perturbed the hierarchy is clear from a recent speech of San Juan's Archbishop Davis in which he castigated "birth controllers and social science experts with a vehement desire to remake a culture."

The Church was further abashed when International Planned

Parenthood Federation's Western Hemisphere Branch chose Puerto Rico as the site for its 1955 meetings. The meetings were picketed and the Association of Catholic Physicians held a simultaneous competing conference a stone's throw away.

The Church's protests were having a marked impact on the Department of Health, when in 1957 an extensive, privately financed family planning program involving major educational services and the widespread distribution of a new contraceptive was instigated. Mrs. Celestina Zalduando, a distinguished public servant who had been Director of the island's welfare department, was named as director, and newspapers announced that the Association for Family Welfare was to be "financed by a St. Louis millionaire . . . with a budget of a great amount of money and will embrace the whole island." This announcement produced stronger than usual invectives from Catholic sources. Mrs. Zalduando was verbally attacked from the pulpits, including that of her own church, and *Juventud*, the Catholic Youth Organization paper, advised her in an open letter, "He who laughs last laughs best, and when you die, you will not laugh." When the testing of a new oral contraceptive was announced as part of the Association's program, *Juventud* likened the "barbarians who crucified Christ" to "those who today crucify Him again with pills."

As early as 1952, on the eve of the election, Bishop McManus gave a preview of things to come when he attacked the Governor and the Popular Party for its pro–birth control policy. After a Popular landslide he asked, "Are not Catholics who gave their votes to his party cooperative in these immoral campaigns?" Although McManus had been very close to the Statehood party and to its leader, Ponce industrialist Luis Ferré, his position found its most sympathetic audience among the *Independentistas*. The Independence Party, which was the only threat to the Populars in the 1950's, espouses complete political independence from the United States, and bases its case more on nationalist sentiment than on economic ideology. Its right wing has been highly nationalistic and anti-American, possessing an almost mystical sense of destiny for the Puerto Rican people. Catholicism is ideologically and sentimentally intertwined with this nationalism, and birth control has tended to be viewed both as genocidal and as anti-Catholic. In 1951 the Union for the Defense of the Moral Law was formed, led by a top-ranking *Independentista*. In addition to making frequent attacks on the government, it petitioned the Puerto Rican constitutional committee to write in prohibitions against teaching and propaganda in favor of birth control, diffusion or sale of contraceptive literature or materials, premarital medical examinations, divorce, and artificial insemination. Although its activities were short-lived, top leadership in the Christian Action Party drew heavily from it and from the Independence Party, both in terms of ideology and personnel.

Catholic efforts have recently been directed largely at the middle class, especially at professionals. The Jesuists sponsor special retreats for elite groups and have "reconverted" a number of influentials. In recent years, for the first time in Puerto Rican history, the Rosary could be heard during lunch in some government offices, it became fashionable to send one's child to a private Catholic school, and a Catholic University began to produce young Catholic intellectuals. The Catholic revival was matched by the formation of a variety of Catholic professional organizations. There now exist associations of Catholic physicians, social workers, nurses, and teachers. The professions, key to a successful birth control program, have been splintered by a division into secular and religious organizations. The latter expend a major proportion of their efforts in combating the birth control program. Representatives from the professional organizations created a Special Propaganda Committee which last year sponsored a televison series entitled "Love, the Source of Life." In these programs, "Neomalthusianism" was attacked by specialists in economics, psychiatry, theology, medicine, and social work.

The public arguments used by opponents of birth control fall into four major categories: birth control is unnecessary, birth control is immoral, birth control is harmful, and birth control is sinful. Since the last argument is straightforward and familiar, only the first three will be illustrated.

Over the last decade articles on the "population question" have abounded. Is Puerto Rico overpopulated? Church spokesmen have favored the theory that it is not overpopulated but economically underdeveloped, and that there is something wrong with a government if it cannot support its people. Even a pronatalist stance has occasionally been taken. *Juventud* recently exhorted Puerto Rican women to "have the children that God wants you to have," and in the town of Vega Baja the priest eulogized a group of women who had had from 15 to 25 children each. In presenting each with a picture of the Holy Family he explained that "we, in celebrating this act, have wished to present to the people of Vega Baja these large families as models of worthy imitation."

This position is not monolithic, however, and along with a pronatalist or laissez-faire approach to births goes an awareness that a lower birth rate might be desirable. If the Ponce diocesan newspaper in discussing problems of family size in 1958 recommended that "humble and simple" Christians rely on "Him who has made no mouth without bread and has a remedy for every ill," they also maintained a year earlier that "the Church does not oblige any couple to have more children than they can bring up." And if Ponce's Bishop recently wrote that "Pure egoism drives government to want fewer people," he could also write a decade ago that "I admit also that a reduced number of births would alleviate the Puerto Rican problem." Despite apparent ambivalence, it is probably safe to agree with Father Dune's appraisal of the situation as voiced in a 1957 *Commonweal* article: "The Church recognizes the need for reducing the present birth rate as well as does the insular government."

When it comes to the means for reducing the birth rate, however, there is no ambiguity. Mechanical and chemical means which divorce the sexual act from its "legitimate end" become an especially vicious kind of hedonism bordering on prostitution.

As put by a writer to *El Mundo*, "We would be sinning if we did not protest against the dishonor which they are bringing to the Puerto Rican woman, against those who try to corrupt and degrade her, taking away the crown of the Christian mother, and making of her the worst which can be said of any woman." Bishop McManus has held that the use of the sex organs only for pleasure amounts to atheism, and others use it as leading to complete social disorganization. Dr. Ibern Fleytas, for example, listed the components of the moral holocaust which might ensue from contraceptive practice: "We would find innocent creatures rushing into free love; prostitution would acquire the force of a whirlwind; and an infinite number of homes would tremble, fearing infidelity. . . . Unbridled instinct would become a beast trying to satiate its appetite on virtue. . . . Who would ever revive the morals of Puerto Rico after they had been torn to pieces?"

Moral degradation is not the only consequence of birth control. In recent years there has been even greater stress on the consequences to the health of the woman. Leading Catholic physicians, psychiatrists, psychologists, and social workers have been hammering home in the press and over television the alleged dangers of contraceptives. In an open letter to the Director of the Puerto Rican Welfare Association, Dr. Ramón Sifre summarized some of the medical arguments against birth control which were aired at the 1955 meetings of the Catholic Medical Brotherhood: "The gynecological aspects were amply discussed by Dr. Rafael Gil, Associate Professor of Obstetrics and Gynecology of our School of Medicine. He proved very convincingly that contraceptive methods may cause illnesses in the genito-urinary tract. . . . Dr. Luis M. Morales, Professor of Psychiatry of the School of Medicine . . . proved to our satisfaction how, when a woman is deprived of something so basic to her being as is her reproductive capacity, severe emotional conflicts arise which can result in the whole gamut of psychiatric illnesses . . . from a state of anxiety to a real psychosis."

In place of contraceptives, Dr. Morales recommended "conjugal chastity, emphasizing the fact that moderation in the satisfaction of all appetites leads to better control of oneself and good mental health."

The deleterious consequences of sterilization have also been outlined. The most impressive list of possible consequences was assembled by Dr. Ibern Fleytas: "Nobody could prove that a sterilized person would afterwards be in normal health. Frequently sterilization results in flatulence, idiocy, premature senility, and a change of sex."

Probably the most ingenious theory can be attributed to a group of five distinguished citizens of Ponce. In a letter to the press, they expressed the view that such illnesses are produced by rebellious sexual organs which turn against those who humiliate them by means of contraceptives. "The very nature of the human body is so rebellious against any moral violations that its very organs, especially the most delicate ones, become strongly vindictive against those who act according to principles contrary to human dignity and the sanctity and unity of the family."

The biggest medical bomb, however, was dropped by Dr. Gil during a March 1959 radio program. With reference to the experiments on an oral contraceptive in Puerto Rico, Dr. Gil, with no apologies to rules of logic, "cited the case of a young patient who after taking the drug for two years, discovered an ovarian cancer." This comment produced a front-page story in *El Mundo* and a banner headline in *El Imparcial:*

CANCER DANGER CITED FOR FEMALES
SUBMITTED TO BIRTH CONTROL

While this particular storm blew over quickly, a much uglier charge and one with deeper roots grew out of the experiments. The notion that continental Americans or the procontinental government of Muñoz Marín were attempting to promote national genocide by means of birth control was promoted by *Independentista* leaders over a decade ago. In 1949 *El Imparcial* referred to "a plan to put an end to the reproductive capacity of the Puerto Ricans," and not long after, the party leader, Concepción de Gracia, condemned the government for "clandestine experiments" in which Puerto Rican women "are being used as guinea pigs in an immoral experiment." Both the anti-"American" and "guinea pig" themes were revived after the announcement of the new birth control association and its testing program. The Ponce diocesan newspaper in attempting to account for the phenomenon of a well-financed family planning program could muster only two hypotheses: "Some say it is the whim of an eccentric millionaire who does not know how to spend his money usefully. Others claim it is a trick on the part of some few Americans who hate the Puerto Ricans, and who want to deter their propagation in order to stop Puerto Rican emigration to the mainland."

With regard to the testing of an oral contraceptive, Drs. Gil and Sifre were quick to ask "the possible reasons for having chosen Puerto Rican women to test this drug . . . when in continental U.S. experimentation of this kind has been principally limited to animals." The Christian Action Party decided to pick up the pill–guinea pig theme in its campaign. In its leaflets it referred to "neo-malthusian projects using an infernal contraceptive pill and using our women as guinea pigs for this abominable experiment. . . . Puerto Rican mothers! How many tears and what dishonor this infernal pill which the materialists are beginning to call the free love pill will bring to your homes!" The Bishops were careful specifically to denounce the pill as "unnatural" and "another form of birth control." A major PAC ad in *El Mundo* features an open letter to Muñoz Marín from a Barranquitas peasant (campesino) as saying, "the Popular Party permits the use of thousands of humble women as guinea pigs . . . that's horrible . . . against the fifth and sixth Commandments."

The position of the opposition parties throughout the controversy was interesting. Muñoz' call to other parties to join him in denouncing the Bishops' pastorals fell on deaf ears. The *Independentista* party, largely drained of its Catholic zealots, maintained silence, but the Republican Statehood Party soon became embroiled. The President of the Party, García Méndez, jumped on a section of the PAC bandwagon and condemned the Popular Party's "irresponsible attitude toward the Catholic Church," its "easy divorce laws," and its "anti-Christian philosophy." On birth control, however, he was mysteriously silent, possibly because PAC had proven not only that his party had been in power when Law 136 was passed, but that García Méndez, himself had been one of the Law's most enthusiastic supporters. On the other hand, Ferré, the Statehood Party's candidate for governor, while holding that the pastoral letter controversy was "strictly a political matter between the governor and three bishops," tried to steal the PAC program away from them. He belatedly came out for repeal of the birth control laws, and in favor of religious education. His conversion to Catholic principles was unappreciated by the PAC who regarded it both with suspicion and as an indication of their own strength. After the election Ferré complained to the *New York Post* that the Bishops' "mistake" helped Muñoz and cost his own party 50,000 votes.

While there seems little chance that Law 136 will be rescinded, there is every evidence that in the past few years Church opposition has eroded away the public program. Physicians in public clinics and hospitals are far more timid than previously about dispensing materials and performing sterilizations.

The defeat of the PAC was a pyrrhic victory for birth control advocates, for what faint heart the government had for family planning was rendered even fainter by the battle. In the years following the election, there was little indication of anything but the most cautious of approaches by official agencies. The private association on the other hand, which had shown bold and imaginative approaches in its first five years (1957–1962), was emasculated in the second five years by the tapering off of funds from its principal donor, understandably disillusioned by the government's failure to take over the program or learn from its experimental efforts in education and services.

Only the shift in United States official policies resuscitated the program during its death throes from economic strangulation in 1966. The Association's executive director announced the award of a half million dollar grant from Washington's Anti-Poverty Program, and indicated optimism that "in some years" her program would be unnecessary. In an interview reported by the *San Juan Star* on June 12, 1966, she stated:

We hope to recruit people on the local level so that the services of the Family Planning Association can be tightly incorporated into the community. Eventually, when we go out of business, when this thing ends in some years, we will at least have left connections between the people and the physicians of Puerto Rico.

Nevertheless, there remains a feeling of uneasiness in the island about longer-range relations with the Church. What worries Puerto Ricans was well expressed in a Catholic postelection brochure: "The Roman Catholic Church counts its age in centuries . . . political parties and their leaders in years. God will have the last word."

8

Haitian Attitudes toward
Family Size

Over the past decade results from studies of attitudes toward family size have been surprisingly similar. When lower-income, poorly educated women are asked for their ideal family size or the number of children they desire, the responses cluster around three or four children. Such surveys have heartened those interested in population control, and have convinced many social scientists that motivational aspects present only minor obstacles to public acceptance of birth control. However, there are a number of reasons for raising questions about highly optimistic conclusions in this regard.

(1) Studies by the writer and his colleagues show that high proportions of the women who state family size preferences also admit that they have never thought about this question before.

(2) Such studies also disclose a high degree of ambivalence about numbers of children. Respondents are able to agree with contradictory statements about family size.

(3) There is some evidence that public and private opinions concerning family size may differ, private opinion favoring small families, public opinion favoring large. Since interviews are characteristically conducted "in private," the opinions elicited may be biased in this direction. Actually, public opinions may be at least as influential as private in predicting behavior, especially in the village culture of underdeveloped countries.

(4) There is also the possibility that the converse of the above

is true, that lower-class respondents may identify middle-class interviewers as having attitudes favorable to small families; and, in an attempt to please, conceal their *private* opinions.

Thus, now that a good deal of ground-breaking substantive work has been done in this area, the pressing need is for methodological studies which will assess the effects of the interviewing situation and the interviewing instruments on responses. Such considerations prompted the writer in 1959 to initiate a small project employing highly unstructured interviewing techniques in relatively primitive conditions.

The study was supported by the Population Council, the Conservation Foundation, and the Cornell Social Science Research Center. The country chosen was Haiti. With over 80 percent of its adult population illiterate, a per capita national product of less than one hundred dollars per year, and with a density of 925 persons per square mile of arable land, Haiti is the most underdeveloped country of the Western Hemisphere.

A village of about 200 families situated 70 miles from the capital city was chosen for study, and a Cornell graduate student of anthropology, William Nibbling, was trained in conducting the interviews. Mr. Nibbling lived for three years in the village and conducted the interviews in Creole after about six months' residence, over a period of three months in 1959.

Three-fourths of the male household heads engage exclusively in farming, and most of the others combine farming with another trade. Even the village elite, the mayor and two judges, work their land with their own hands. Only 9 percent of the female household heads or the wives of household heads are economically inactive, 40 percent engaged exclusively in agriculture, the remainder combining agricultural work with the marketing of produce or small-scale retailing.

The modal years of education for adults of both sexes is zero, (41 percent for male heads and 65 percent for their spouses), but those who have had any school at all are relatively well educated —a median of five and a half years for both sexes with almost a quarter of the educated males having had nine or more years of schooling. The average household has 4.6 members. Ninety-one percent of the village household heads are Catholic, one percent Protestant, and the others claim no religion.

THE INTERVIEW

A major difficulty inherent in poll-type questioning techniques is that the very raising of the question structures the response. Thus, although a person may never in his life have considered the question of an ideal number of children, when specifically asked in these terms, a numerical reply can easily be made. In the present instance a method was desired which would encourage the respondent spontaneously to articulate attitudes on family size, and which would answer the following general questions: (1) Does the subject *perceive* families in terms of size, that is, is the concept of number of children salient? (2) Does the subject prefer a larger or smaller family? (3) Does the subject perceive any connection between the number of children and the economic status of the family?

A series of photographs of four different Haitian families was designed in which two characteristics were systematically varied —number of children and economic status. The small families contained a man and woman and three children, the large families a man and woman and six children. In the well-to-do families the subjects wear shoes and are relatively well dressed. In the poor families the children are either naked or in rags, and the adults poorly dressed. By combining the two characteristics, four photographs are created: (1) The small well-to-do family; (2) the large well-to-do family; (3) the small poor family; and (4) the large poor family.

The photographs were presented to the subjects in pairs (the sequence of pairs being randomized), and three general questions asked, ranging from the unstructured "Tell me about these two families," through the more specific "Do you see any differences between them?" to the most specific "If you were given the choice which would you prefer to be, the (man) (woman) in this family or in this one?" (Because the attention span of the subjects was limited, only certain combinations of photographs were used: For questions of *differences* between the families, photographs 1 and 2 were presented together, and photographs 3 and 4. For questions of *preference*, the sets compared were 1 and 2; 3 and 4; 2 and 3; and 1 and 4. It will be noted that in all four comparisons the size characteristic is varied, while economic status is varied in only two.)

Interviews were conducted with 44 males and 45 females, chosen from 191 censused families which contained a conjugal pair. In order to get equal numbers of common law and married couples the sample was stratified for marital status. In terms of education, occupation, and size of landholding, the sampled groups are practically identical with the remainder of the village families. Because of the oversampling of common law couples, however, the sampled cases are slightly younger and have given birth to about one child less than the nonsampled families.

Initial Reaction

After a period of small talk and after an effort to secure a minimum of privacy the photographs were introduced as follows:

I would like to show you some photos of Haitian families. A friend of mine took these pictures in another village far from here. Everybody sees something different with the families in these pictures. I would like to have your own ideas. Let us look at these two families first.

The most frequent initial response was a mixture of delight and confusion. Little accustomed to photographs of any kind, the respondents often immediately reacted with exclamations of pleasure or amazement. This was soon followed, however, by a rather extended period of silence, the respondents often at a loss for what was expected of them.

Madam K had no initial response to the photos. She looked at the first set and did not know what to say. She would look at the pictures and then look at me during the pause. Finally, I had to start with the first question to get some kind of response.

Although she tried hard to be cooperative, as are nearly all informants, she was confused by the presentation of the pictures. At the start she did not know what was expected of her. Asking the question: "Tell me about these two families" did not sufficiently channel her reaction into significant channels.

Even after a more specific probe asking, "Do you see anything different between the two families," as many as 20 subjects on the first set and 19 on the second failed to make a response or could not cite a difference. The responses of those who did cite differences were classified into three categories: differences in family size, differences in economic or social status, and differences in other characteristics. Rather surprisingly, differences in size of families were mentioned only by a minority of those who responded. (See Table 12.)

While about three-fourths of the respondents cited economic differences between the families on each of the two sets, only

Table 12. Percent who cited size, socioeconomic, or other differences, photo sets 1 and 2 (percentages are based on those who cited a difference)[a]

Differences	Set 1	Set 2
Size	35	39
Socioeconomic status	78	73
Other	30	42
Number	(69)	(66)

[a] Percentages total more than 100 because some respondents cited differences in more than one category.

just over a third mentioned size. Of the total sample, including those who failed to note any differences at all, only 11 percent mentioned a difference in size on both sets, and an additional 34 percent on one set. Thus, the majority mentioned size on *neither* set. Indeed, factors extraneous to the design were mentioned as frequently as size. These included the skin color of the individuals in the photographs, the facial characteristics, the general appearance of the children, the pose of persons in the photographs, and so on.

We were particularly interested to discover whether the characteristics of those subjects for whom the family size seemed more salient were different than those for whom it seemed less salient. The subjects were therefore divided into those who failed to mention size differences on either set of photographs (49 cases), those who mentioned it with respect to one set (29), and those who mentioned it for both sets (10). These three groups were then compared on age, education, sex, marital status, size of landholding, socioeconomic status, and number of births.

There are virtually no differences between those who made no mention of size and those who mentioned it on one of the two photographs. Those who mentioned size differences on *both* sets of photographs surprisingly are more likely to be males, somewhat older, and of less education. Because of the very small number in this group, however, even these differences are not significant. In short, whatever salience on family size does exist seems to be more or less randomly distributed among the population of the village.

Preferences

On all four sets of photographs, the subjects were asked to choose whether they would prefer to be the man or woman in one family or in the other. Again, about a quarter of the respondents failed to make a selection. In this case they would say either that they liked both of them, disliked both of them, or, more frequently, that they simply could not choose between them. In addition to possible confusion concerning what was being asked, there appears to be a tendency against making invidious comparisons on religious grounds.

I can't make a choice. It's the work of God whether one is poor or well off. How can I say that I choose one or the other?

I don't prefer one over the other because both families are children of God. . . . God makes all people.

I can't choose because God makes all men. He makes some poor and others rich.

Among those who did articulate a choice (see Table 13), there was a decided tendency to choose the larger family. Of the 50 respondents who made a choice on all four sets of comparisons, only 4 percent chose the small family in all instances, 12 percent in three out of four, 26 percent in two, 34 percent in only one instance, and 24 percent in none. A total of 67 persons made at least three choices, and of these almost two-thirds chose the large family three or four times out of four, while only 18 percent chose the small family three or four times out of four.

The most popular photograph was of the large well-to-do family. It is preferred by three-fourths of the subjects, whether compared with a small poor family or a small rich one. It is also apparent that when economic level is held constant (sets 3 and 4), the larger family is preferred by most. In the most extreme comparison, where the small family is well-to-do and the large one is poor, only half chose the small family. There is some evidence suggesting that subjects perceived the large well-to-do family as higher in socioeconomic status than any other family, due to certain unintended cues in dress and household furnishings. This could mean that economic level was not in fact held constant. Even assuming this to be the case, the conclusion to be reached from Table 13 is either that there is a bias toward the

Table 13. Choice of large or small family, four paired comparisons

Comparisons	Percent who failed to make choice	Percent of choosers preferring small family	Number of choosers
Small well-to-do with large poor	24	50	(68)
Small poor with large well-to-do	17	23	(74)
Large poor with Small poor	26	38	(66)
Small well-to-do with large well-to-do	24	22	(68)

large family, or that family size is not highly relevant to the choices made. We can pursue this question further by examining the reasons given for the stated preferences.

(1) Economic reasons are given more frequently than reasons of size, even when economic level was presumably held constant. Of those giving reasons for their choices (ranging from 73 to 89 percent), those citing economic factors range from 36 to 44 percent over the four sets; those citing number of children range from only 9 to 31 percent. However, it should not be assumed that all these economic reasons refer to the superiority of the well-to-do families. Of those who preferred the poor families, over a third did so precisely because they were poor. There was, first of all, a positive identification with the poor family.

Because he is like me, poor.

I like this one. When I am working in my garden, I am in the same form.

I like her because it is a poor family. If I knew them, I could give them a little gift.

Because I am poor too.

The lower class has a number of rationalizations for the superiority of the poor, chief among them being that they are the children of God.

God loves poor people . . . because they think of God often . . . but when they are rich, they don't think of God. They forget Him. They have money. They have an auto; they drive to H.; they drive here and there . . . and God likes children too.

If you are poor, you know many people, and if you are rich, you don't know many.

Not only are the poor the children of God, but there is the corresponding belief that riches may be attained by a compact with the devil. This will be discussed subsequently.

(2) While size is almost twice as likely to be mentioned when the economic level is held constant than when it varies, economic factors are mentioned by similar proportions regardless of variation in size.

(3) The most striking finding is that the most frequent reason given for choices was in terms *neither* of size nor economic status, but in terms of other, "extraneous" considerations. Over the four sets of choices, such reasons were cited by 57 to 65 percent of the respondents. Moreover, in just over half of the cases citing preferences, reasons falling in this general category were given *exclusively*; that is, were unaccompanied by reasons in the size or economic category. Given below are examples of the kind of comments made which were classified as "other."

I prefer this one. The picture is taken better.

She has a pretty face.

Her head is down.

She stands better.

He seems to be more docile.

We have seen that the poorer family was often preferred since the poor are viewed as the children of God. Similarly, the large family was occasionally chosen specifically since the larger number of children were seen as a gift of God.

Even though he is poor, God has given him many children because he has faith in God. God helps him.

God gives poor people many children and rich people he gives money instead of children. [I wonder why?] I don't know. [Then, addressing herself to me and to the neighbor]: Don't you always see poor people with a lot of children? [Neighbor vigorously agrees, while I take refuge in writing.]

He is poor but God has given him many children. . . . They are a gift from God.

(4) Only a minority of those who prefer the large family mention size as a reason for their preferences. (The range is from 9 to 28 percent over the four sets.) Moreover, in three out of four sets, those who prefer the large family are no more likely to mention size than are those who prefer the small one. (When the small well-to-do family was compared with the larger well-to-do, only 15 of the 89 cases preferred the small. Almost half of these, however, did so because of its small size. Among those who chose the larger family, less than a quarter did so for its size.) Upon completion of the paired comparisons, respondents were asked four open-ended questions: (1) How do you think it came about that some had few children and some had many? (2) Why was one family better off than the other? (3) Could they have done anything to keep from having many children? and (4) What do you think is the best number of children for a person in your circumstances?

Responses to these questions underscore the low salience of family size already discussed, and, to a certain extent, help to account for it. Dealing with the last question first, we find that

62 persons, or 7 out of every 10, say that this is a matter entirely up to God. The most frequent kind of response is illustrated below:

I can't know that. It's what God desires to give me.

I can't tell you because that's up to God.

What God gives me, I will accept . . . I will say thank you God for as many children as He gives me.

Other responses show even more clearly the apparent absence of any norms or ideals as regards family size. Neither the large nor small family is preferred; any number which God sends is the right number.

If God gives me ten I would be happy. If He gave me two I would be happy too. . . . God gives the poor people many children.

What God gives me. I made eight children and lost six. If He gives me more I will say thank you.

If I have ten children I will say thank you. If He gives me only four or five I will say thank you too, and if He gives me none I will say thank you.

If God gives me two I would be happy. If He gave me 100 children I would be happy too, because that is not for me to decide.

If He gives me ten that is all right, and if He gives me one that is all right too.

One can infer from such statements that ten children is viewed as a large family, and that three or less is probably viewed as a small one. But it is perfectly clear that one ought not to prefer one or the other, being grateful rather for whatever God chooses. It is interesting, however, that the few people who did state a preference named a small family. The median number preferred by the twenty individuals stating a number was 2.4. Only one person gave a number higher than 4. Apparently, if a person can break away at all from the stereotypic "whatever God sends" he goes all the way and prefers a small family.

In any event, the norm is an avoidance of mentioning an ideal number. One possible explanatory key is provided by responses to the other three questions. In the first place, conception is viewed as something beyond the control of man, and almost exclusively in the hands of God. When asked why some couples have few children and others have many (question no. 1), only 19 percent gave responses other than "the will of God." Among the 19 percent, a third ascribed it to the age at marriage and the most frequent other response referred to natural differences in fecundity, with a few scattered references to child mortality or to the farming out of children. While this initial question was intentionally somewhat vague, question number 3 was pointed directly at the possibility of deliberate human intervention ("Could they have done anything . . . ?"). Even here, 14 percent did not know and 65 percent said no. Most of those who gave a negative response put the matter squarely in the hands of God.

No, people cannot do that because it's God who makes children.

I don't think that's true, because God gives children.

No, people can't do anything to not make children because it is God who gives them children.

Just as deviation from poverty was sometimes explained in terms of magic so deviation from having children was ascribed to evil forces by some respondents.

An evil air prevents a woman from making a child. It contaminates the child in her stomach and she cannot give birth. It is an evil spirit that takes the child.

There are some who make magic to kill children. Married people don't do that but unmarried people.

Most of those who said people could do something to inhibit fertility, however, referred either to abortion or to vague "medicines," or to "injections" given by doctors.

They can go to a doctor and he gives them medicine. . . . I think he can give the wife an injection. I don't know exactly. . . . If people want only two or three children they can do it. But actually it is God who does all things.

They say you can go to a doctor and he gives the woman an injection so she can't make children . . . but that's against God if she is not sick.

Only one respondent, the wife of a farmer, described by the field worker as an "agricultural innovator" mentioned mechanical or chemical means of contraception, and only one woman (the mistress of a relatively well-to-do villager) expressed any interest in contraception.

Most respondents flatly denied that anyone but God could control fertility, and showed no interest in the matter. More persons than those who actually admitted it probably have heard that "something" can be done, but the knowledge is so sketchy and so contaminated by ideas of black magic, abortion, and evil motives that it is not normally mentioned.

Fatalism

The one dominant theme which runs through the interviews regardless of the subject being discussed, is the importance of God and fate in the determination of human events. This is brought out most clearly in answer to the question, "Why was one family better off than the other?" Of the 85 people who could answer the question, 40 attributed the difference solely to God, and 24 attributed it to luck or destiny (usually in terms of one's star). We have already seen that the complete compliance with God's will kept a significant minority from making a choice between the families. Such a choice would indicate dissatisfaction with one's lot in life.

I don't know (why one family is better off). It's God who gives such things. . . . He chooses one family to give much to and another to give little. That's His affair. If a family has a fortune, we can't be jealous of that, because that's God's work.

Indeed, to break out of one's divinely assigned niche is so unlikely that it requires supernatural action. To do so by one's own efforts therefore requires an allegiance with the powers of darkness.

Informant seemed to be saying that one's course in life was determined at the moment of birth but that one can change it by resort to magic. He can go to a bocor who tells the men to do certain things and the man will then make money. . . . There was agreement from the people present. He said that one could get ahead by work but only to the limited extent of supplying basic needs for his family. If one's lot was to be poor, then even work would never make him well off, let alone rich.

The man gets money of the devil. . . . It works but it's bad for the man. It's evil.

If this is the major theme, it is also true that an important minor one is present: 19 respondents cited naturalistic explanations for the discrepancy in wealth; 13 of these referring to harder work, the balance to greater capacity, intelligence, education, or inheritance. These same respondents were also much more likely to mention economic differences between the photographs in which we had intended *no* economic differential. Close to half of this group cited such differences on each of the two sets which "controlled" for economic status, while only a quarter of the other respondents did so. Thus they are *highly sensitive* to cues indicating socioeconomic status. Further, twice as many in this group as in the main group stated a preferred family size (and we recall that this tended to be small), and 42 percent of them (as opposed to only 15 percent of the others) said something could be done to determine the number of children one has. Since they seem, then, to be a rather select minority with relatively modern attitudes, let us look more closely at their characteristics (see Table 14).

Table 14. Comparative characteristics of those with supernatural and those with naturalistic explanations of economic success

Characteristics	Supernatural	Natural	Contingency coefficient
Percent of households with wife employed in a nonagricultural occupation	32	61	.56[a]
Percent of households with husband employed in nonagricultural occupation	17	35	.44
Percent with "large" landholdings	21	44	.49
Percent married	49	87	.74[b]
Median age of wife	29	38	—
Median years education of household heads	5.1	7.5	—
Number of cases	(69)	(19)	

[a] Chi Square significant .05.
[b] Chi Square significant .01.

Those who gave naturalistic explanations for the economic superiority of one family over the other tend to come from the elite households of the village: the husbands are better educated, are larger landholders, and are more likely to engage in non-farming occupations on a part- or full-time basis. They are also older and more likely to be married, the latter characteristic perhaps reflecting this social status. In short, they are the minority of villagers who are more experienced, wiser, and more successful.

CONCLUSIONS

The results of the present investigation are in marked contrast to those in other underdeveloped areas, where women, in response to poll-type questions express an interest in a small number of children. The projective technique revealed that family size is a matter of very low salience for most of the Haitian men and women interviewed, that norms concerning the appropriate family size seem nonexistent and inappropriate for most subjects, and that an attitude of religious fatalism about number of children is characteristic. The beginnings of a more modern orientation toward the world generally are present among a minority of the older, better educated, and more well-to-do villagers, but this does not seem as yet to have materially affected their basic views on the matter of family planning.

While our original purpose was to determine whether a different manner of questioning would produce different kinds of responses, we must regard the foregoing results with caution. Unlike the usual poll-type inquiry, the investigator lived in the village and conducted the interviews over an extended period of time. As a non-Haitian white he may have been associated in the minds of the villagers with the only other person of this category in the village—the French priest. The investigator was, in fact, a close friend of the priest's, although he carefully avoided attending religious services. On the other hand, the priest reported that he never discussed the Church's position on family planning with parishioners because it was unnecessary—they did not know enough about it to be interested or to be tempted. Nor, he reported, was this matter discussed in other villages of Haiti. Of course, even though explicit attention to birth control is absent, more general values on resignation to one's fate may well be inculcated by the Church. Information on this point is lacking. The field worker reports his feeling that even if the *source* of such attitudes is religious, they are by now genuinely held by the villagers who were not merely paying lip service to a philosophy they did not necessarily share.

An equally plausible explanation for the present findings would be that Haiti is different from other areas of the world as regards attitudes toward family size, and that the same kind of responses would have been elicited by poll-type interviewing. The safest conclusion to be reached from the present findings is that they are challenging enough to justify replication and extension. The projective technique should be applied in areas where polling methods have been or are being used, and poll-type techniques should be tried out in Haitian villages.

9

The Caribbean Fertility Studies

Over the past decade two major investigations concerning fertility control among lower-income classes have been completed in the Caribbean area—one in the Commonwealth of Puerto Rico, the other in Jamaica. Both are small islands of roughly similar topography, climate and population size; both historically have been colonial-agricultural areas with heavy reliance on African slave labor, and both are currently exhibiting high birth rates and low death rates. Their small size, internal cultural homogeneity, and demographic position made them ideal as laboratories for investigation. Moreover, while the islands are sufficiently similar to make comparison meaningful, they are sufficiently distinct culturally (Spanish *vs.* British) to make comparisons fruitful. Each investigation involved a three-stage design moving from relatively broad and unstructured techniques and concepts to highly refined experimental approaches, and from more theoretical to more applied concerns.

Exploratory or pilot stage. In Puerto Rico 72 rural and urban couples, and in Jamaica 99 rural and urban wives and a subsample of 53 husbands, were given unstructured interviews ranging in length from two to six hours.

Verification stage. Based on results from the pilot investigations, larger-scale sample surveys were carried out, using shorter interviews with questions more amenable to statistical analysis. In Jamaica an area probability sample of 1,400 currently mated urban and rural women was employed. In Puerto Rico a similar representative sample of the island's household heads was employed for questions on knowledge and use of birth control, but the interview proper was given to 888 wives and 322 husbands, drawn from the out-patient case loads of health centers and prematernal clinics on the island.

Experimental stage. In an effort to determine whether educational methods can affect knowledge, attitudes, and behavior in the area of family planning, experimental designs were set up. Matched or experimentally varied groups were exposed to varying educational treatments and the results compared with non-treated control groups. In addition to the pre-experimental interviews, Jamaican cases were reinterviewed six weeks, one year, and three years after treatment. Puerto Rican groups were reinterviewed six weeks and one year later. In Puerto Rico pamphlets and group discussion techniques were separately assessed, as well as varying educational contents. In Jamaica, case visits were added as a third educational technique, but the content was roughly identical in all treatment groups.

Finally, in order to establish a kind of base line, a third area was chosen for pilot investigation. This is the island of Haiti, where levels of poverty and illiteracy are considerably higher than in the other two islands. In this instance, entirely different techniques of investigation were employed in a rural village.

On the basis of the various studies, we can draw up three necessary and three facilitating conditions for effective fertility control.

NECESSARY CONDITIONS

The necessary conditions are (1) ends or values which explicitly favor a family size less than is normally achieved without control; (2) awareness of the means of achieving family limitation; (3) acceptability of the known means.

Each of these conditions can be seen as varying on a continuum, and both individuals and societies can be assigned a position on any of the three measures. The apparently simple model is complicated by the fact that various combinations of scores could theoretically produce family planning behavior, and by the fact that the scores are probably interrelated. For example, even in the absence of knowledge of all currently popular forms of birth control, if the ends were of sufficient intensity, individuals or groups could resort to infanticide or abstinence from sexual relations, techniques known to all populations but usually disapproved. On the other hand, a highly acceptable and simple method such as an oral pill, especially if sugar coated, might be taken despite quite weak motivation. Moreover, while high motivation might produce a search for knowledge, the simple provision of knowledge might precipitate motivation among peoples who know of very few means of control.

Since populations in underdeveloped areas generally fall toward the negative end of the continuum on our three necessary conditions, we have added three "facilitating" conditions that make adoption of family planning much more likely.

FACILITATING CONDITIONS

Distribution of Means

While methods such as coitus interruptus, abstinence, and to some extent abortion and rhythm are theoretically available to all individuals in all societies, the accessibility of mechanical, chemical, and surgical techniques varies enormously from society to society, and between classes and social groups within a given society. Presumably, the less accessible are such techniques, the higher the motivation required to initiate and persevere at effective family planning.

135

Social Organization

While any number of social organizational characteristics can facilitate or impede adoption of family planning, we refer here mainly to the extent to which the family structure implements the development and sharing of goals and knowledge which its members may possess individually. The degree to which the sexes are segregated both outside and within the family, the patterns of dominance in the household, the stability of conjugal bonds, the norms concerning cross-sex discussion of intimate topics, and the articulation of the family with other social institutions, are among the aspects relevant to the adoption and preseverance of family planning activity.

Salience

Here we refer to the priority of limited family size in a hierarchy of values. It might appear that a high priority is a necessary condition. While this may be the usual case, it is plausible that even among a population where family limitation has very low salience, such methods as reversible sterilization or a periodic injection or oral tablet might be adopted.

As a means of organizing our Caribbean research in summary fashion, we shall more or less impressionistically assign a +, o, or +o (indicating a mixed or intermediate situation) to each of

Table 15. Position on scales of necessary and facilitating conditions for effective fertility control, three Caribbean islands

Conditions	Haiti	Jamaica	Puerto Rico
Ends	o	+	+
Awareness	o	+o	+
Acceptability	o	+o	+o
Distribution	o	+o	+
Organizational facilitation	?	o	o
Salience	o	o	o

the six conditions for each of the three societies studied. As seen in Table 15, the Haitian village falls at one end of the continuum, Puerto Rico at the other. However, while Haiti approaches the theoretical limits in one direction, Puerto Rico falls short of the limits in the other direction.

JAMAICA

There is little question that Jamaican women generally prefer small families. When the 1,400 women were asked how many children they would like if they could live their lives over, 76 percent said four or less children, and only a negligible proportion said this was up to God or fate or that they did not care. Moreover, when asked whether they wanted more children, 80 percent of those with four or five children and 84 percent of those with six or more replied negatively.

Nine out of every ten women said they believed there were "people who do something to keep themselves from having too many children," suggesting that the population is aware that human intervention in the course of fertility is *possible*. When it comes to specifying the means, however, it is clear that knowledge is inadequate. For example, 16 percent of the urban and 40 percent of the rural women were unable to name a birth control method. Of those who could, a fifth of the responses were either very vague or referred to magical techniques. While *recognition* of methods named or described by the interviewer was higher, it is still the case that only a third of the rural women (but 73 percent of the urban women) had a good knowledge of even the best known method, the condom. No female method was well known by more than 10 percent of the rural women.

The ignorance of techniques is partly due to the lack of contraceptive services. At the time of writing, the entire city of Kingston was serviced by one private clinic, and only one parish had a network of rural clinics.

Attitudes toward birth control are mixed. A direct question on general approval or disapproval evokes approval from half, disapproval from just over a third, with the remainder ambivalent or undecided. That this is partly based on ignorance of birth control or unfavorable connotations of the term itself is indicated by the fact that when asked whether they would take a pill once a month to keep from "making a baby," 70 percent replied affirmatively. Moreover, the greater the knowledge of specific methods of birth control, the more positive the attitude.

In terms of family organization, marital relationships are probably more equalitarian than in Latin societies, and the culture is less restrictive concerning discussion of sexual matters between husband and wife. In this sense, the social organization is favorable to joint planning and responsibility for family limitation. But in a more important sense, the structure inhibits both fertility and fertility control. About three-fourths of Jamaican births occur out of wedlock, a product both of common law and of relatively transitory sex relations which can be termed "visiting." In our sample, 29 percent of the women were married, 44 percent were living in common law unions, and 27 percent in visiting relationships. The nonlegal relations are quite unstable. Thus, half of the women 35–40 had had three or more unions, and only a quarter had had only one union. Largely as a consequence of nonexposure time between unions, the average woman evidences a considerably lower fertility than would be the case if unions were stable. Moreover, motivation for family planning is greatest among the unmarried couples, since women in this status have some misgivings about bearing illegitimate children, while married women feel that bearing children is especially appropriate to their status. Motivation for family planning is therefore inversely related to the degree of stability of the relationship.

This motivation refers to *women*, however. Males are less concerned about family planning, especially in the least stable relations, partly because they can relatively easily escape the burdens of child support by desertion. Consequently, although the situation is mixed, we have assigned a zero value to family organization because the fluid nature of the unions creates such diverse motivations on the part of male and female that action is generally inhibited.

A good indication of the lack of salience of the whole issue is given by the fact that only 38 percent of the women report ever having discussed the number of children they want with their mates. Even among those who have had five or more births (and over 80 percent of these want no more children) only 32 percent have discussed the matter. Those who want no more children are no more likely to have discussed their concern than those who do.

Obviously it is difficult for the matter to become salient if there is only a vague awareness of the means for solving the problem. In this connection it is of interest that there is a positive correlation between knowledge of birth control and discussion of family size preferences.

In the light of the inadequacy of knowledge, poor family organization, and low salience of family limitation, it is not surprising that only 7 percent of the rural and 17 percent of the urban women have ever tried a birth control method.

PUERTO RICO

Puerto Rican women favor especially small families. Over three-quarters of the women expressed a preference for three or fewer children. When asked whether they wanted more children, less than 5 percent said they did not care or it was up to God, and after three or four living children about nine out of every ten want no more.

Puerto Ricans are relatively knowledgeable about birth control. As many as a fifth of rural women with no education know six or seven methods. Rural males with no education know an average of 3.3 methods. The condom and sterilization are the best known, diaphragm and jelly the least known. Even here, however, knowledge is surprising. A quarter of all household heads and 17 percent of rural household heads of no education knew of the diaphragm.

Attitudes toward birth control are generally favorable. When asked, "Who has the right to use birth control?" only 15 percent of the women said no one or only those whose health is in danger. Two-thirds said they would advise their daughters to use birth control, and 85 percent of those who have never used a method said they would take a contraceptive pill if available.

To a certain extent the superior knowledge and favorable attitudes of Puerto Ricans are due to the fact that a full range of contraceptive materials and sterilization have been available in government clinics for the past two decades.

As we have seen, however, the clinics have never been used to any great extent, and when asked where their wives could obtain free birth control materials, only 22 percent of the uneducated rural males could answer (the proportion rises to about 70 percent for those with some high-school education). Although 41 percent have ever used a method, only 19 percent of the national sample have ever used a mechanical or chemical method. Of those who have ever used birth control, a quarter have used sterilization only. Including sterilization, about a third are currently using some form of birth control. Use of nonsurgical methods tends to be erratic and ephemeral.

Thus, despite a desire for small families, relatively good knowledge of methods, favorable attitudes, and an excellent public system of clinics, family limitation has not yet "caught on" in the same sense as in modern industrial societies. Presumably this is a matter of "time." Nevertheless, there is reason to believe that the lag between facilities and effective adoption of birth control practices may be to a large extent due to the absence of a family organization conducive to effective family planning, and to the relatively low salience which the issue of family planning has for most Puerto Rican families.

As we have noted, questions of birth control are infrequently discussed among Puerto Rican couples. The consequences of this are at least twofold. First, in the absence of effective communication each of the mates makes assumptions about the other according to cultural stereotypes. In static cultures this mechanism may be satisfactory; but in a society undergoing rapid change, the stereotypes may be quite out of tune with reality. For example, according to our investigations, husbands attribute more modesty (a cultural ideal) to their wives than their wives actually possess, and wives assume greater virility drives and desire for children than their husbands actually possess.

Second, knowledge about contraception is not pooled. Thus, whereas close to nine out of every ten males learned about a contraceptive method prior to marriage, over 40 percent of the women learned about their first method some time after their second pregnancy. Comparing over 300 couples, in only a fifth of the instances did the husband and wife know the same number of methods. In a third of the cases the husband knew more methods than his wife, and in about half the instances the wife knew more than the husband. In short, many of the positive attitudes and much of the knowledge possessed by Puerto Ricans individually fail to affect behavior because they are not exchanged in a group situation—in particular within the conjugal relation.

Perhaps another reason for this is that the whole issue of family planning does not yet have high salience for Puerto Ricans. While birth control is both possible and permissible within the culture, it is not culturally *prescribed*. Thus, while facilities are present and attitudes are generally favorable, there is no institutional pressure or even encouragement to use such facilities. And while Puerto Ricans generally prefer small families, there are also cultural values which emphasize the contrary. As a result we find a high proportion who can agree with a statement favoring small families, but also agree with its exact opposite. Without strong institutional supports, the issue does not become salient until specific individual pressures make it so. Such pressures occur only after the couple has had several children. Thus, for families in which the household head is 40 or older and has ever used birth control, the practice was not initiated until after an average of 3.6 pregnancies for those with less than nine years of education, and after 2.9 for those with nine or more years of school. But without prior experience with birth control and without institutional reinforcement, contraceptive practices then tend to be erratic, ineffective, and consequently short-lived. In this context, the unusual popularity of female sterilization in Puerto Rico is explicable; but a large proportion of these occur beyond the point at which a major impact on the birth rate could be made. Sixteen percent of the women in a national sample of households were found to be sterilized, and this accounted for half of all methods currently in use. Sterilized women who have been married for ten or more years had had an average of 6.6 pregnancies in their last union. About half of the sterilized women had had prior contraceptive experience. The low salience produces late starting, which produces the need for an easy but foolproof method.

EXPERIMENTAL PROGRAMS

From our experimental programs we can learn the extent to which educational techniques can precipitate contraceptive behavior among more or less "ready" populations such as Puerto Rico and Jamaica. In both instances the programs were remarkably successful considering the brief educational exposure. In Puerto Rico 42 percent of those given pamphlets and 31 percent of those who attended group meetings had used birth control six weeks after treatment. Although the impact was considerably less six weeks after treatment in Jamaica, after nine months 40 percent in the urban areas and 21 percent in the rural areas had used birth control. A number of general conclusions can be drawn from these studies.

(1) Such short exposure programs are effective in precipitat-

ing contraceptive behavior among a substantial minority, but are less successful at maintaining it. Of those who had started contraception in Puerto Rico six weeks after the program, about half had discontinued a year later. In Jamaica a fifth of the urban and close to a third of the rural users had stopped using a year after treatment.

(2) Almost *any* stimulus which makes the issue salient and puts it in a public context of approval by respected groups will precipitate use among that minority psychologically ready. This conclusion is supported by at least two facts: (a) Pamphlets are about as effective as the more intensive group or individual case approach. In Jamaica, none of the three methods was markedly more successful than others, and in Puerto Rico, pamphlets were somewhat more successful than group methods in getting people to start practicing contraception. (b) Even the control groups responded positively, presumably as a consequence of the interviews alone. In Puerto Rico a quarter of the control group and in Jamaica a fifth of the control cases started birth control subsequent to one or two interviews. Despite the objectivity of the interviews, six out of every ten women in the Puerto Rican control group (as opposed to eight out of every nine in the treatment groups) said they had benefited from the interviews, and of these a quarter said they had learned about birth control methods and close to half said the interview made them think about having a small family. The interviewers were well educated and middle class, the respondents poorly educated and lower class. The mere fact of such "authorities" raising questions about birth control and family size, we believe, increased the salience of the issue and gave it some institutional support.

(3) For *sustained* contraceptive behavior, and perhaps for reaching the large hard core who do not respond at all, more intensive type programs would seem required. It is of interest in this connection that in Puerto Rico while pamphlets were somewhat more effective in getting families started, group meetings were more effective in sustaining contraceptive practice, once it

had begun. In Jamaica, although meetings were somewhat more successful among the initially most favorably disposed cases, among others no method was outstanding.

What practical conclusions stem from these findings?

(1) Pamphlet materials have far more efficacy than previously supposed among populations processing a certain degree of literacy and predisposition to family limitation. Indeed they are *particularly* effective among such populations since they are not already saturated with other printed media. Thus, in Puerto Rico, 83 percent of the women who received the pamphlets reported that they had read them, and recognition tests largely support the validity of their statements. In Jamaica, all the urban women and eight of every nine rural women reported reading them. Most of the remainder said they had the pamphlets read to them.

(2) Group meetings, in addition to their great expense in time, personnel, and money, suffer the great disadvantage of attracting only the most highly motivated. In Puerto Rico, despite very great efforts at insuring attendance, only 16 percent of the women and 8 percent of the men attended all three meetings. Fifty-nine percent of the women and 40 percent of the men attended at least one of the three. In Jamaica, where only one meeting was held, 46 percent of those invited attended. I would propose that these limitations be turned to advantage. Pamphlets can easily be distributed to the entire population. Meetings should be employed *only* for the opinion leaders in the community, for those most highly motivated, and for those already practicing contraception. The meetings could then serve a dual function—to *sustain* and *reinforce* by means of explicit group and institutional support, the motivation and behavior of those already started, and to form a small, highly motivated elite which could stimulate others in the community by means of the normal person-to-person channels of verbal communication.

(3) *We do not know* what, if anything, is especially effective in motivating the hard core which failed, by and large, to respond to any of our educational treatments. Even the intensive case

visit approach did not appear especially effective. In the absence
of further research I would recommend two minor and one major
course of action. First, that this group be reached by means of
pamphlet materials; second, that where feasible such materials
stress sterilization, abortion, coitus interruptus, and oral tablets.
By and large, however, the group which represents from half to
three-quarters of the populations, should be *ignored* in any explicit fashion, the principal ammunition being directed at opinion
leaders and "contraceptive leaders."

HAITI

The immensity and impracticality of other alternatives is
vividly illustrated by our case materials on Haiti, a culture which
we have scored o on each of the six conditions for family limitation. As shown in Chapter 8, there is no cultural ideal concerning
the appropriate number of children for villagers, and when asked
why one family had few children while others had many, almost
three-quarters said such things were determined by God or
chance.

A key to the Haitian situation was provided by the question:
"Why is one family better off than another?" Seven percent said
they did not know, and 70 percent said it was sheer luck or good
fortune sent by God.

When one's general lot in life is determined by vague forces
extraneous to the individual, and when numbers of children are
viewed in the same context, there is simply no solid foundation
on which to build a program of family limitation. The only hope
lies in raising educational levels and economic opportunities to a
certain minimum point at which self-improvement seems both
possible and desirable. Indeed, it is precisely at this point that
general programs are most needed and make most sense. At one
end of the continuum, population control programs are impracticable, at the other end largely unnecessary. Societies such as

Puerto Rico and perhaps Jamaica are in the intermediate stage, where educational levels and economic development have reached a point at which educational programs in the family planning sphere can help to precipitate *some* of the necessary conditions, but do not have to work in a complete vacuum. *Without* such programs, these societies may eventually reduce their fertility to modern levels; but our Caribbean studies indicate that such natural processes will be tortuous, slow and uncertain.

10

Social Class and Preferred Family Size in Peru

In 1960 and 1961, with the financial assistance of the Population Council and the collaboration of the Peruvian School of Social Work, about 2,000 currently mated women in the city of Lima, Peru, and several hundred women in the highland town of Huaylas were administered a questionnaire on fertility and attitudes toward fertility.[1] (Data on Huaylas occasionally will be introduced for contrast with Lima, but the small number of cases and skewed distribution of social class there prevent detailed breakdowns.) Interviewers were instructed to categorize the respondent's social class in one of four ranked groups, depending on a list of criteria provided by a Peruvian commercial research firm. In the urban area, 13 percent of the sample was placed in the highest class (A), 25 percent in class B, 38 percent in class C, and 25 percent in class D. Although the judgments were largely subjective, differences among the classes in education, expenditure, occupational distribution, and so on are marked (Table 16).

As regards occupation and household appliances, a very decided gap appears between classes B and C. Educational variation is more regular. Whereas 73 percent of the class A women have

[1] For details concerning sampling and interviewing in Lima, see Chapter 15. For contrast with the capital city, the highland town of Huaylas was chosen; and 344 women, representing the total eligible population who could be contacted, were interviewed.

Table 16. Objective class-related measures, according to interviewers'
appraisal of social class (in percent)

Objective indices of class	Class A	Class B	Class C	Class D
Husbands with white-collar occupations	87	69	15	4
Wives with less than four years' education	0	2	33	68
Households with refrigerator	99	71	8	1
Households with television	85	59	9	1
Number of cases	(253)	(490)	(757)	(495)

finished high school, for example, the median years of school for
the other classes is 9.0, 5.2, and 2.9.

A basic question to be answered by this survey was the extent
to which class differentials exist in fertility and attitudes toward
fertility. From Table 17 it is evident that there is an inverse rela-

Table 17. Live births by social class

	A	B	C	D
Age standardized mean	2.6	2.8	3.7	4.6
Index numbers (Class A = 100)	100	108	142	177
Women 40–44	3.8	4.3	5.3	7.2
Index numbers (Class A = 100)	100	113	139	189

tion between class and fertility, but, similar to the pattern in
Table 16, differences between the two upper classes are small.
Moreover, while the three highest classes are clearly limiting
their fertility by some means, this may not be the case for class
D. As a crude point of comparison, in 1940 the average *mother*
aged 40–44 living outside of Lima-Callao had had only 6.1 live

births according to the census. Thus, in 1960 the average class D urban *wife* was having one birth more than nonurban mothers had in 1940.

Table 18. Number of children preferred, by social class and residence

Number of children	Lima				Huaylas
	Class A	Class B	Class C	Class D	
0–2	8	17	29	31	22
3	17	18	13	15	11
4	37	30	24	18	12
5–6	26	24	22	21	21
7+	7	6	8	9	12
All God sends	4	3	3	4	13
No answer	1	2	1	2	9
Total	100	100	100	100	100
Mean no. preferred[a]	4.6	4.3	4.1	4.0	5.1
Mean no. preferred, standardized for no. of living children[b]	4.7	4.4	4.0	4.0	5.1
Median no. preferred for daughter	4.1	4.0	3.3	3.2	3.6
Number of cases	(253)	(490)	(757)	(495)	(344)

[a] Eight or more preferred children scored as 9; "all God sends" scored as 10.

[b] Standardized by the distribution of living children for the entire Lima sample.

Table 18 shows the distribution of responses to the question, "If you were to live your life over, how many children would you like to have in all?" Medians are also given for responses to the question, "How many children would you like your daughter to have?" As might be expected, Huaylas stands out in the number of children considered ideal, with a quarter of the women wanting seven or more, and with a mean desired number of five. Within Lima, however, we see a *direct* relation between class and preferred number. Despite the fact that there is also a direct relation between preferred number and actual number of living children, standardizing for the number of children does not diminish the differences between classes in the desired number of children. A similar relation prevails with respect to the number desired for one's daughter. No less than 46 percent of the women in the lowest class would like their daughters to have two or fewer children, whereas only 9 percent of the upper-class women prefer such a small number of children for their daughters.

Since lower-class women want fewer than the upper class but in fact have more, it is not surprising to find that a third of the lower-class women have already exceeded the number they consider ideal, as contrasted with only 12 percent of the upper class.[2] If the respondents are consistent, we would then expect that the lower class would be less interested in having more children than they now have. This turns out to be true, as measured by a direct question on whether or not additional children are desired (Table 19). At every parity from one to six or more living children, the lower-class women are less likely to want additional children. Even when age and parity are simultaneously controlled, the class difference holds up in most instances. It is also of interest that age and parity are independently

[2] These figures are derived from direct cross-tabulations of the exact ideal number with the exact number living. The discrepancy is apparent at all parities; e.g., for women with less than four children, only 4 percent of the lower-class but 13 percent of the upper-class women have at least one more living child than they consider ideal. For women with five or more children the corresponding figures are 40 and 64 percent. These findings are in marked contrast to those found for a group of several thousand Israeli maternity cases, where "less than 3 percent admitted a preference for some number smaller than the number they already had" (R. Bachi and J. Matras, "Family Size Preferences of Jewish Maternity Cases in Israel," *Milbank Memorial Fund Quarterly*, XLII [April, 1964], 45).

related to the desire for more children, controlling class. A similar pattern holds for the median preferred number of children (not shown), except that the relation to age is no longer a consistent one. In short, we find a persistent tendency for lower-class women to prefer fewer children than upper-class women.

This finding, while contrary to popular stereotypes about the lower classes in Peru, is entirely plausible. Urban lower-class aspirations for education and material acquisitions may not differ greatly from those of the upper classes, but their ability to achieve them is far less. Thus, 98 percent of classes A and B said they wanted, and 96 percent said they expected, their youngest female child to have a secondary-school or university education. Class C has about the same desire (93 percent), but their expectation drops off sharply to 71 percent. In class D the discrepancy is even larger: 71 percent desire secondary-school education but only 48 percent expect it. Figures for male children are virtually identical. (In Huaylas, aspirations and expectations come together at a *low* level—15 percent and 12 percent.) The gap between desired and *achieved* education for children is doubtless even greater. In such a situation, children are a greater disadvantage to the lower than to the upper classes.

While this may be so objectively, what evidence do we have that it is so perceived by the lower classes? To what extent are the class differences in desired family size due to the perception of the *economic* disadvantages of children? To answer this question we asked whether having an additional child would affect the family's economic situation, and if not, whether having three more would affect it. The same type of question was asked with respect to the effect an additional child would have on the respondent's health. ("Do you believe that having one more child would harm, improve, or not affect your health?")

For present purposes, the significant finding is that there is a marked difference between classes with respect to the question on economic impact but not with respect to health. When child parity is introduced, lower-class women with less than two

Table 19. Desire for more children, by social class, age of mother, and number of living children, Lima

Age of mother	Percent who want no more children		Bases for percentages	
	Classes			
	A, B	C, D	A, B	C, D
0–1 living children				
20–29	2	14	123	155
30–34	7	21	28	34
35+	31	29	32	38
2–3 living children				
20–29	15	32	114	260
30–34	30	33	96	99
35+	50	54	137	93
4+ living children				
20–29	40	58	20	140
30–34	36	54	55	166
35+	62	73	138	265

children are more likely than upper-class women to indicate that an additional child would affect their health adversely. But for two children or more, there is no difference between the classes. On the other hand, for the effect on the economic condition of the family, at each parity from two to three times as high a proportion of lower-class as upper-class women answered the question affirmatively.[3]

Table 20 gives a more comprehensive summary of the re-

[3] Only 14 percent of upper-class women with two living children think an additional child would affect their economic situation, and this figure does not vary as the number of children increases. On the other hand, 23 percent of the lower-class women with two living children report that an additional child would affect their economic situation, and the proportion increases steadily to 39 percent of those with six or more children.

sponses to the economic question by combining information referring to both one more and three more children.

Table 20. Mean economic sensitivity score, by number of living children and social class,[a] Lima

Living children	Classes A-B	Classes C-D
0	1.6	2.2
1	1.9	2.6
2	2.4	2.7
3	2.3	2.9
4	2.4	2.9
5	2.5	2.8
6+	2.1	3.0

[a] Respondents were scored from one to four depending on combinations of responses: 1 = neither one nor three more children would affect the economic situation; 2 = three more children would affect it a little; 3 = three more children would affect it a lot; 4 = one more child would affect the economic situation.

At each child parity the economic sensitivity of lower classes to additional children is higher than that of the upper classes. Moreover, while the sensitivity increases with a fair degree of regularity as parity increases among lower-class women, the trend is less clear for upper-class women; those with six or more children are no more sensitive than those with two. In short, differences revealed between social classes in desired numbers of children are consistent with differences in concern over the *economic* impact of additional children.

But to what extent does the perception of economic and health disadvantages of additional children predict the actual desire for more children? People might believe children a financial and health disadvantage and still desire more because of other advantages. Or they might feel no economic or health disadvantages and still want no more children. Table 21 shows that

Table 21. Percent who want no more children, by opinion about impact of an additional child on health and economic situation, Lima

Economic situation	Health would be harmed	Health would not be harmed
Would be harmed	90	73
Would not be harmed	64	48

there is indeed a relation. If an additional child is felt to harm both the economic and health situation, then in nine out of ten instances in Lima the woman will want no more children. However, the absence of such feelings does not guarantee that a woman desires more children; half of those who feel no economic or health disadvantages still do not want any more children. Put another way, 46 percent of those not wanting more children feel that neither their health nor economic situation would be affected by having an additional child. This might suggest that motivations other than these are of considerable importance—for example, the amount of energy required to rear children, or a sense of inappropriateness about having "too many" children. Since 95 percent and 61 percent of the two upper classes but less than 5 per cent of the lower classes have servants, it is clear that the former are far less concerned with energy loss due to additional children than are the lower classes.

We have seen that women in the lower classes want fewer children than the upper classes, but in fact have more. There is, of course, a long and complex chain between felt desire for a particular number of children and its achievement, and we obviously cannot expect to discover all the intervening mechanisms in this particular analysis. However, the attitudes toward numbers of children that we have been discussing can be of various kinds. For example, when a middle-class American woman says she wants no more children or that an additional child would cause economic difficulties, the likelihood is that she has given

154

the matter a good deal of thought, has discussed it with her husband, knows what to do about it, knows what her friends are doing about it, and so on. We believe that the same statement from a lower-class Peruvian woman does not generally imply any of these things, and may imply only a *latent* interest in controlling family size which at the moment of the interview may represent little more than wishful thinking.

Several types of data support this conclusion. Thus, when women are asked, "Have you ever thought about the number of children that you would like to have, or haven't you thought about it?" the proportion who answer positively drops markedly with social class: 73 percent in the top class, 62 percent in class B, 42 per cent in class C, and 35 percent in the lowest class. In Huaylas the comparable figures are 23 percent and 16 percent for the upper and lower classes. Moreover, among those who have thought about it, lower-class women are much less likely than upper-class women to have discussed it with their husbands, the percentage dropping from 87 in class A to 57 in class D and 49 in Huaylas.[4] Notwithstanding the fact that lower-class women readily responded to our questions on desired numbers of children and wanted fewer children than upper-class women, only a minority say they have ever thought about it or discussed it with their husbands. Moreover, in Lima the more children a woman has the less likely she is to report ever having thought about it. Both class and parity independently affect the relation, so that as many as 90 percent of the class A women with one birth or none, but only 29 percent of the class D women with five or more births, ever thought about the number of children they wanted. While it might be thought that the parity relation in fact conceals a relation with age, Table 22 shows that in most

[4] This does not impede women from specifying their husbands' desires. For example, in the lowest class, despite the fact that only a fifth of the women have ever discussed the number of children they and their spouses want, 93 percent answered a question asking how many more children the husband wanted.

Table 22. Percent who have ever thought about
number of children wanted, by social class, number
of living children, and age of mother, Lima

Age of mother	Number of living children		
	0–1	2–3	4+
Classes A and B			
20–29	79	71	65
30–34	86	69	56
35+	77	64	49
Classes C and D			
20–29	56	40	33
30–34	41	44	34
35+	47	54	29

instances women under 30 are no more likely to have thought about it than women 35 and over.[5] Class and parity, however, still maintain their relation to thought about ideal size.

Since we did not collect data on contraceptive practices, we cannot test the most plausible hypothesis: that those who think about family size are more likely to attempt to control it.[6] Of special interest here, however, is the fact that unlike our previous attitude-items on family size, thought and discussion about family size show a positive relation to social class and a negative relation to fertility.

Thus we noted that desire for more children decreased and sensitivity to the economic implications of additional children increased with greater number of children, but thought about the matter diminishes. In fact, there is no relation between ex-

[5] In the Israeli study, where only 40 percent reported ever having considered the desired number of children, a marked negative relation to parity and little relation to age were also found. Bachi and Matras, *op. cit.,* p. 40.

[6] This proved to be the case in Puerto Rico and Israel. See R. Hill, J. M. Stycos, and K. W. Back, *The Family and Population Control* (Chapel Hill: University of North Carolina Press, 1959), pp. 317–18; and Bachi and Matras, *op. cit.,* p. 48.

pressed attitude toward the number of children and whether or not the matter has been discussed or thought about (Table 23).

Table 23. Attitudes toward family size by previous thought and discussion, classes C and D,[a] Lima (in percent)

	Three more children would not affect economic situation	Three more children would not affect health	0–3 children preferred
Discussed number desired	17	40	42
Thought about but didn't discuss number desired	15	36	42
Have not thought about number desired	18	38	45

[a] The same absence of relation exists among the two upper classes.

The fact that most lower-class women have not thought about family size and that there is no relation between desire for few children and thought or discussion about it leads to questions concerning the meaning of expressed attitudes on family size. The consistent preference among the lower classes for smaller families regardless of the measure utilized and regardless of age or parity suggests that the responses are not random. However, we believe that, because the degree of factual information about fertility and birth control is so limited and distorted for the lower classes, attitudes favorable to the small family remain in a latent stage, perhaps largely unrealized by the respondent until articulated to an interviewer.

In 1960, such topics were not discussed in the mass media in Peru, nor are they a part of public health services. Since the lower classes have little access to private physicians or scientific literature, we wished to assess their knowledge of general facts concerning fertility and mortality. As we can see from Table 24, it is clear that most lower-class women in Lima do recognize the existence of differential fertility in Peru—that rural and poor women have more children than do urban and rich women. Most of the Huaylas women, on the other hand, are ignorant of differential fertility and of changes in fertility and mortality. In Lima, with the exception of differential fertility, there are significant proportions misperceiving important social facts, and this misperception is inversely related to social class. Thus, as we move toward the lower class, increasing proportions believe there has been no change in fertility in the past generation; and of those who do see a change, over a third of the lower-class women believe fertility has *increased*. It might be thought that this is the result of perceptions of reduced infant mortality which make contemporary families seem larger. However, we see that lower-class women are also less likely to believe there has been a change in mortality, and, among those who do, over half of the two lower classes believe there has been an increase in mortality. (According to pre-test data, this is because they feel that the air, food, and life in general were more healthy in the "good old days.") Moreover, those who say fertility has increased are somewhat less likely to say that mortality has declined.

Another interesting finding is that lower-class women believe the average woman bears ten or eleven children. In our own sample, currently married women aged 40–44 in the lowest-class group had an average of 7.2 live births. Census data for 1940 recorded only 6.1 live births for mothers 40–44 living outside the Lima-Callao area. Thus, lower-class women are greatly overestimating the fertility of the average woman.

Finally, lower-class women are less likely than upper-class women to believe other women desire the same number of children as they themselves do. Of those who see a difference, the lower classes are much more likely to think other women want *more* children than they. Thus lower-class women are more

Table 24. Perceptions concerning fertility and mortality

	Lima				Huaylas
	Class A	Class B	Class C	Class D	
Percent who say poor have more children than rich[a]	75	88	94	89	29
Percent who say rural women have more children than urban[b]	90	92	82	74	21
Percent who see no generational change in fertility[c]	16	11	22	36	64
Percent of remainder who believe fertility has increased[e]	5	7	18	38	47
Percent who see no generational change in mortality[d]	19	18	22	29	66
Percent of remainder who believe mortality has increased[d]	20	37	56	59	30
Median births by age 55 attributed to other women[e]	6.5	8.2	10	11.4	10.1
Percent who believe other women want same number of children as respondent[f]	53	47	37	37	51
Percent of remainder who believe other women want more children than respondent[f]	14	20	34	35	54

[a] Do rich women have more children, fewer children, or the same number of children as poor women?
[b] Do women from the country have more, fewer, or the same number of children as women from Lima?
[c] In your parents' generation, did women have more, fewer, or the same number of births as nowadays?
[d] In your parents' generation, did more, fewer, or the same number of children die as nowadays?
[e] How many births have most women had by the time they are 55 years old?
[f] Do other women want to have more, fewer, or the same number of children as you?

likely to believe that other women want more children and have more children than they do.

CONCLUSIONS

We initially raised questions about lower-class motivation with respect to family size. It was found that lower-class Lima women desire fewer children and are more sensitive to the economic implications of additional children than are upper-class women with the same number of children. Moreover, in absolute terms, preferred family size is moderate; half of the women want no additional children after they have had two.

Further questions were raised about the significance of verbal statements of preference in a social context where the topic is not generally a public one and where the society does not support in a normative or technological sense the realization of such ideas and preferences. It was found that only a minority of lower-class women report they had ever thought about the number of children they desired, and even fewer had ever discussed it with their husbands. The preference for only a few children is probably a latent one which is brought out by the interviewer's questions but which seems to have little significance for behavior.

In the absence of a social context in which information on family size and family size goals is shared, a number of erroneous beliefs are current which further serve to inactivate small-family preferences. Lower-class women greatly overestimate the average fertility of other women, suggesting that they must think of their own fertility as quite low. Similarly, much more so than is true for women in the upper classes, they believe other women desire more children than they do. They are also much more likely to believe that both fertility and mortality have increased since their parents' generation. Lower-class women are, however, generally aware that differential fertility exists between social classes and residential groups. Most of the generalizations hold in an even more exaggerated form for the rural women.

The implications for applied programs are that, while lower-class urban women do not have to be convinced of the general desirability of having a moderate number of children, they need to have their latent inclinations activated by shifting discussion of the whole matter into socially approved channels. In addition to technological information, they must learn that other women want small families, that their own fertility is not lower than that of others, and that mortality as well as fertility has declined. Most of all, they must be encouraged to think about and articulate private opinions about family size until public opinion is created. A program that emphasizes not the creation of new goals but the social implementation of latent ones should have unusual appeal in urban Latin American societies that are typically conservative about public programs of fertility control.

11

Contraception and Catholicism
in Latin America

Catholic resistance to "artificial" means of birth control and a tendency on the part of Church leaders to extol the large family are among the explanations frequently advanced for high rates of fertility in Latin America, as well as for justifying pessimistic outlooks for the future of fertility in Latin American cultures.[1] Recent studies in the United States have left little doubt that both religious affiliation and religiosity are important factors in fertility.[2] Summarizing the results of their study of metropolitan mothers, Westoff and his associates write: "Religious preference . . . is the strongest of all major social influences on fertility. Catholic couples want the most and Jewish the fewest children, with Protestants in an intermediary position. . . . Catholics by and large appear to want larger families and they have them."[3]

---

[1] The attitudes and behavior of Latin Americans with respect to the family planning issue are also of great importance to the course of Catholicism itself. One of every three Catholics now lives in Latin America, and in another forty years every other Catholic may be a Latin American.

[2] The relation between religiosity and fertility variables in the United States is less clear for non-Catholics than for Catholics. See Gordon F. De Jong, "Religious Fundamentalism, Socio-Economic Status, and Fertility Attitudes in the Southern Appalachians," *Demography*, II (1965), 540–48.

[3] C. F. Westoff, R. G. Potter, and P. C. Sagi, "Some Selected Findings of the Princeton Fertility Study: 1965," *Demography*, I, No. 1 (1964), 133.

The "Growth of American Families Study" of the mid-fifties also found strong relations between the degree of Catholicism and both attitudes and behavior. For example: "Catholics who seldom or never attend church are more likely to be users (of birth control) than are other Catholics."[4] "Catholic wives who attend church regularly expressed unqualified disapproval [of birth control] in just about twice the proportion for those attending seldom or never."[5] "Whether they approve of the practice of family limitation or not, Catholic wives still expect more births than Protestant wives."[6]

On the other hand, the relevance of Catholic teaching for fertility has recently been challenged by Day, who maintains it "will be a factor leading to higher fertility among Catholics only when (a) there exists a high level of economic development, and (b) Catholics constitute a numerically and politically important, but not dominant, *minority* of the population."[7] In most of the countries in Latin America, Catholics satisfy neither of these conditions. An early study in Puerto Rico produced findings consistent with Day's hypothesis in that non-Catholics appear to be no more liberal (with respect to birth control, ideal family size, etc.) than Catholics.[8] But when the minority hypothesis was specifically tested in Protestant Jamaica (West Indies), about the same results were obtained as in Catholic Puerto Rico.[9]

[4] R. Freedman, P. K. Whelpton, and A. A. Campbell, *Family Planning, Sterility and Population Growth* (New York: McGraw-Hill, 1959), p. 107.

[5] *Ibid.*, p. 159.   [6] *Ibid.*, p. 284.

[7] L. H. Day, "Catholic Teaching and Catholic Fertility," Paper 202, *Proceedings of the 1965 World Population Conference* (New York: United Nations, 1967). Day has a useful bibliography of studies of differential Catholic fertility.

[8] J. M. Stycos, K. W. Back, and R. Hill, "Contraception and Catholicism in Puerto Rico," *Milbank Memorial Fund Quarterly*, XXXIV (April 1956), 9.

[9] J. M. Stycos and K. W. Back, "Contraception and Catholicism in Jamaica," *Eugenics Quarterly*, V (December 1958).

While the Caribbean studies of Catholicism could not be extrapolated to Latin America, a series of surveys has been conducted in Latin American cities within the past few years, making it possible to duplicate the earlier analyses in a variety of Latin American settings.

We have already mentioned, in Chapter 4, the Peruvian study conducted by the author and the CELADE series conducted in Bogotá, Buenos Aires, Caracas, Mexico City, Panama City, Rio de Janeiro, and San José.[10] In late 1964, a similar survey was conducted in San Salvador, sponsored by the Salvadoran Economic Planning Committee and the Cornell International Population Program.[11] Data from these surveys form the basis of this chapter.[12]

[10] The Peruvian study is described in Chapters 10 and 15, the CELADE surveys in Chapter 4, and in J. M. Stycos et al., "The Cornell International Population Program," *Milbank Memorial Fund Quarterly*, XLII (April 1964). For preliminary results of these surveys, see C. A. Miró, "Some Misconceptions Disproved: A Programme of Comparative Fertility Surveys in Latin America," in B. Berelson et. al., eds., *Family Planning and Population Programs* (Chicago: University of Chicago Press, 1966), and C. A. Miró and F. Rath, "Preliminary Findings of Comparative Fertility Surveys in Three Latin American Cities," *Milbank Memorial Fund Quarterly*, XLIII (November 1965).

[11] See C. J. Gómez, *Estudio Económico y Social de la Familia del Area Metropolitana de San Salvador*, El Salvador: (mimeo., 1965); and "Religion, Education and Fertility Control in Latin American Societies," Paper 471, *Proceedings of the 1965 World Population Conference* (New York: United Nations, 1967).

[12] In the case of Lima we shall rely primarily on an unpublished term paper by Dario Menanteau, "Religion as a Factor in Attitudes and Fertility Behavior in Peru" (Cornell, 1964); and for Salvadoran data on the papers by Gómez. In assembling the data on the other six cities, the writer was assisted by several students as part of an informal seminar of the International Population Program: Robert Gochfeld, Elizabeth Johnson, Enrique Pérez, Haifaa Shanawany, Alan Simmons, and Robert H. Weller. Data from the Buenos Aires study had not arrived at the time this report was prepared.

THE PRACTICE OF CATHOLICISM IN LATIN AMERICA

"The Catholicism of Latin America," according to Father J. P. Fitzpatrick, "has characteristics of its own that generally baffle the outsider. . . . It ranges from an intensity of practice and devotion that is heroic, to an indifference that is difficult to conceive."[13] It is the variation in intensity of practice which we shall emphasize here—variation among Latin American cities and variations among individuals within the same city.

According to recent data, there are more than twice as many priests in the United States than in all of Mexico and Central America. Whereas the United States has 2,500 Catholics for every priest, South America has 4,285 and Central America 6,771.[14] Among the countries which concern us here, the variation in sacerdotal density is considerable, from 3,500 inhabitants per priest in Colombia, to 8,300 in El Salvador.[15] As shown in Table 25, the country rankings differ somewhat, depending on whether diocesan or "religious" priests are considered. However, whatever the measure, Colombia is at one end of the range and Brazil, Panama and El Salvador are at the other.[16]

[13] Cited by L. Gross, "The Catholic Church in Latin America," *Look*, October 9, 1962.

[14] *Statistical Abstract of Latin America* (U.C.L.A., 1962), Table 10; U.S. data apparently refer only to diocesan priests.

[15] Y. Labelle and A. Estrada, *Latin America in Maps, Charts, Tables: Socio-Religious Data (Catholicism)* (Mexico, D. F.: Center for Intercultural Formation, 1964).

[16] By dividing into deciles the range between extreme values for eight religious variables, Alonso creates a five category index for classifying Latin American countries according to their religious structure. Of the countries we are considering, Colombia is in the top decile in seven out of eight measures and is placed in category 1. Costa Rica is in category 2; Brazil, Peru, Mexico, and Venezuela in category 3; and El Salvador and Panama in category 4. None of the countries discussed here fall in category 5, "least religious structure." Labelle and Estrada, *op. cit.*, pp. 269–82.

Table 25. Population (in hundreds) per ecclesiastic, selected Latin American countries, 1960

Countries	Per priest	Per diocesan priest	Per religious priest	Per nun
Colombia	35	61	81	10
Costa Rica	45	85	97	19
Venezuela	50	118	88	21
Mexico	54	69	246	18
Peru	58	140	99	27
Brazil	64	158	107	23
Panama	64	248	86	32
El Salvador	83	166	166	44
Latin America	53	108	103	20

Source: Yvan Labelle and Adriana Estrada, *Latin America in Maps, Charts, Tables: Socio-Religious Data (Catholicism)* (Mexico, D. F.: Center of Intercultural Formation, 1964), pp. 89, 161.

Turning to our survey data, we find a rough correspondence between the parishioner-priest ratio and the religious observance of mated Catholic women in the capital cities (Table 26). Thus Bogotá and San José, where two-thirds of the women report they go to Mass every Sunday, are situated in the countries with the lowest parishioner-priest ratio. With respect to the practice of Communion the range is again from Bogotá, where half the women take Communion at least twice per year, to Rio where only a quarter do so.[17]

[17] Catholic investigators have also noted the nominal nature of Catholicism in Rio de Janeiro. In a study of religious practices in the *favelas,* 84 percent declared themselves to be Catholics, 46 percent were classified as "indifferent to the faith," 38 percent were classified as traditional or folkloric in their practices (practicing only on Christmas, Holy Week, etc.), 7 percent as irregular practitioners, and only 9 percent as regular practicers of their religion—attending Sunday Mass and observing their Easter duty. "A Umbanda Impera Nas Favelas do Rio," *Revista Eclisiastica Brasilera,* June 1958, cited in J. E. Betancur and L. Garcia de Sousa "Current Population Changes in Latin America and the Implications for Religious Institutions and Behavior," *Catholic Sociological Review* (Spring 1959).

CONTRACEPTION AND CATHOLICISM

For purposes of this paper we shall distinguish three gradations of religious observance according to frequency of receiving Communion. The first group will be termed "nominal" Catholics, defined as those women who declare themselves to be Catholics but who fail to receive Communion once a year—a minimum requirement of the Catholic Church. Among the six cities in the CELADE series, the lowest proportion of "nominals" is found in Bogotá (19 percent), the highest in Rio (56 percent). Caracas, Mexico City, Panama City, and San José show 38, 46, 52 and 39 percent, respectively. The second group will be designated as "marginal" Catholics, those who achieve but do not exceed the minimum standard; that is, they attend Communion only once per year. The third group, here termed "devout," receives Communion twice a year or more frequently. The proportion of "devouts" for each city is given in Table 26. Since there is a tendency for education to be positively related to religious behavior (Table 26) we shall hold education roughly constant by classifying our three religious types according to whether or not they have completed primary school. Such a procedure may on occasion clarify the anamolous findings sometimes reported on the relation of religiosity to fertility-related variables.[18]

In seeking to ascertain the relation between religious practices and fertility, we should distinguish between attitudes and behavior. With respect to attitude, we shall distinguish between attitude toward family size and attitude toward contraception; and with respect to behavior we shall distinguish between contraceptive behavior and actual fertility. These distinctions are important since it is possible that religiosity affects one variable or set of variables without affecting others. For example, devout Catholics might want small families but have large ones because

[18] For example, in a survey of women in a working class area of Santiago, Chile, Requena tabulated the outcome of 2,617 pregnancies. "Results of this tabulation were totally unexpected," he writes. "The risk of induced abortion clearly increases with the frequency of Church-going. We have no explanation for this finding." M. Requena, "Social and Economic Correlates of Induced Abortion in Santiago, Chile," *Demography*, II (1965), 42.

Table 26. Attendance at Mass and practice of Communion by educational level

City	Number of mated Catholic women	Percent who attend Mass weekly			Percent who take Communion more than once per year		
		Total	<Primary school	≥Primary school	Total	<Primary school	≥Primary school
Bogotá	1522	68	62	75	49	45	52
Caracas	1251	34	24	43	29	23	35
Lima	1995	49	39	65	—	—	—
Mexico City	1527	60	56	63	30	27	33
Panama City	1330	41	24	48	32	23	40
Rio de Janeiro	1491	27	22	32	24	22	25
San José	1261	67	62	71	24	22	25
San Salvador[a]	1647	—	58	67	—	—	—

[a] Data include non-Catholic women and refer to monthly attendance at religious services. Educational categories refer to "less than six years of education" and "more than six years of education." See Gómez, op. cit.

they do not wish to practice contraception. On the other hand, they might favor large families and disapprove of contraception because of Church teaching, but practice it out of a sense of economic necessity. Their fertility level might reflect this ambivalence, depending on the intrinsic efficiency of the methods chosen, and the consistency with which they are used.

ATTITUDES TOWARD FAMILY SIZE

"Somehow," says Westoff, as if mystified, "the large family as a value seems to become idealized in the culture of a Catholic College."[19] Surely both Catholic education and formal religious observances put one more in tune with Catholic teaching. While disclaimers of a Catholic Church "doctrine" on large families are heard increasingly, there is no escaping the fact that the large family has been idealized by the highest Church authorities and an unknown number of parish priests and nuns. In the contemporary period, Pope Pius XII made many statements throughout his long reign which left little doubt that large families should be a goal of the Christian family and accepted joyfully as a gift from God. A few of his pronouncements are illustrated below:[20]

[To newly-weds (1940):] Look about you, and you see numerous spouses who are full of joy and courage because they are blessed with a charming and abundant flock of children. May you also follow their example.

[To the College of Cardinals (1947):] Fidelity to the laws of God brought the blessing of a rich crown of children. . . . only true heroism . . . is capable of keeping in the hearts of young married people the desire and joy of having a large family.

[To the Italian Association of Large Families (1958):] You represent large families, those most blessed by God and specially loved

[19] Quoted in the *Princeton Alumni Weekly*, April 20, 1965.
[20] Papal citations are taken from A. Zimmermann, *Catholic Viewpoint on Overpopulation* (New York: Hanover House, 1961), pp. 192–206.

and prized by the Church as its most precious treasures . . . to accept joyfully and gratefully these priceless gifts of God—their children—in whatever number it may please him to send them. . . . Large families are the most splendid flower-beds of the Church.

Even Pope John on occasion lauded the large family, cautioning the faithful in 1960 not to be "afraid of the number of your sons and daughters. On the contrary, ask Divine Providence for them, so that you can educate them for their benefit, for your own honor in later years, for the great welfare of your fatherland, and for the eternal homeland toward which we are tending." Surely such widely publicized statements from the leader of the Church must have had their impact on the stance of the parish priest, if not directly on the attitudes of parishioners.

In addition to direct exhortations from the pulpit or confessional, literate Latin Americans are also likely to be exposed to the influence of the secular press, which often extols the virtues of the large family. Three examples appearing in the Mexican press within a period of a few months can be cited.

A feature article against birth control: "Should we destroy the Monument to the Mother? Should we not offer homage to those women who have distinguished themselves by their fertility?"[21]

A father of fourteen, including quadruplets, is extolled for his stand against family planning in a four-column story: "I will have all the children God sends," he is quoted as saying. "I would like to have more."[22]

A feature story, with pictures, of the winners of the "1964 Extraordinary Award for Fertility" (Premio Extraordinario de Natalidad, 1964): "The couple, married 15 years and with 15 children . . . believes that when the public sees . . . the advantages of a large number of children, many couples will follow their example. 'Are you planning to have more children?' we asked. 'All that God wishes!' they replied."[23]

[21] *El Universal Gráfico*, April 8, 1965.
[22] *Novedades*, April 13, 1965.   [23] *Novedades*, March 5, 1965.

In an effort to ascertain the family size norms of Latin American women the following question (with slight modifications in Lima and San Salvador) was asked in all the cities under discussion: "If you were to start a family now, how many children would you want?" Only small percentages in each city replied that this was "up to God" or "as many as God sends," and the overall totals reflect moderate family size goals. There is considerable variation among the cities, from a low of 2.4 for mated Catholic women in Rio de Janeiro to a high of 4.1 for the corresponding group in Mexico City (Table 27). While there is little correspondence between the overall city rankings on ideal size and general religiosity, in all cities except Panama ideal size rises with degree of religious observance, among the better educated women. The trend is less marked but also apparent among the less educated women in most of the cities.[24] In four of the cities there is also a negative relation between ideal size and education holding religiosity constant.[25]

[24] This positive relation between ideal size and religiosity was also observed in the Santiago survey, the mean ideal number of children rising steadily from 3.7 among those who never attend Mass, to 5.0 among those who attend more than once per week. L. Tabah and R. Sammuel, *op. cit.* Recent surveys in Madrid also indicate "a positive relation between ideal size of the urban family, socioeconomic status and religiosity." Women who practice their religion "with little regularity" express a median ideal of 3.0 children, while those who practice "with great regularity," prefer an average of 3.5. See J. Diez Nícolas, "Status Socio-económico, Religión y Tamaño de la Familia Urbana," *Revista Española de la Opinión Pública*, December 1965. That the relation between religiosity and family norms is stronger among better educated Catholics has been noted in American studies. Freedman states that "the attitude favoring moderately large families among Catholics is more influential among the better educated than among the less educated." Freedman *et al., op. cit.,* p. 286. In discussing the rather large family norm among Catholics, Westoff and associates conclude that "a Catholic education is one of the social mechanisms supporting such a norm. It seems to operate primarily at the college level, to some extent at the secondary level, and not at all at the elementary school level." Westoff *et al., op. cit.,* p. 133.

[25] For a discussion of a different finding see Chapter 10.

Table 27. Median ideal family size[a] by education and religious practice

City	Total	Less than primary school			Primary school or more		
		Nominal	Marginal	Devout	Nominal	Marginal	Devout
Bogotá	3.7	3.5	3.6	3.9	3.3	3.7	4.0
Caracas	3.6	3.8	3.6	3.8	3.5	3.3	3.7
Lima	—	3.7			3.6		
Mexico City	4.1	4.5	4.4	4.9	3.7	3.9	4.1
Panama City	3.3	3.7	3.9	3.7	3.5	3.6	2.8
Rio de Janeiro	2.4	2.2	2.6	2.5	2.2	2.3	2.9
San José	3.8	3.5	4.2	4.4	3.4	3.7	4.1
San Salvador[b]	3.9	3.7			5.1		5.4

[a] In computing the median, the class limits for each digit were chosen so that a whole number (2, 3, 4, etc.) would fall at the midpoint of the interval. Open-ended categories such as "as many as God sends" were included at the high end of the continuum in calculating medians. The method for computing medians in the San Salvador study is not specified, and the medians of 5.1 and 5.4 for the better educated women probably reflect computational errors, since they are both implausible and inconsistent with other data in the same table from which they were drawn. See C. Gómez, "Religion, Education and Fertility Control," op. cit., Table 1.

[b] Religiosity categories distinguish between women attending church services once a month or more, and those attending less frequently. See note [a], Table 26.

That these rather general ideals are also reflected in more immediate and specific family size goals can be illustrated by the pattern of responses of women in Lima, Peru, to the question, "Do you want to have any more children than you now have?" Among the less educated women, after the first child there is a small but consistent tendency for the more religious women to want more children at each parity; among the better educated women, the difference is considerably greater.

In the case of Peru we can refine our measure of religiosity by adding the dimension of marriage, dividing the various groups into those who were married in a church service and those who were not. (Most of the latter women are living in

Table 28. Attitudes toward family size, by education, attendance at religious services, and type of marriage, Lima, 1960 (extremes only)

Family size	Primary school or less		Secondary school	
	Weekly Mass and Catholic marriage	Less than weekly Mass and no Catholic marriage	Weekly Mass and Catholic marriage	Less than weekly Mass and no Catholic marriage
Median ideal number of children	4.3	4.0	4.6	3.4
Percent of women with 0–2 living children who want more children	58	54	74	46
Percent of women with 3 or more living children who want more children	28	15	45	28
Number of women	(314)	(327)	(454)	(52)

consensual unions.) Addition of this item further emphasizes the large family orientation of the more religious women (Table 28). As before, differences are sharper among the women with some secondary school education, but are also apparent among the less educated. Better educated women who attend services weekly and were married in the church prefer over one child more than women of a similar education who attend services less frequently and who did not marry in the church. Controlling for numbers of children, the more religious women are much more likely to prefer additional children. (Values for the intermediate types, not shown in the table, fall between the extremes.) While secondary-school educated women who were neither married in church nor attend services regularly are significant for our analytic purposes, we must keep in mind that they are scarce indeed, representing only about 3 percent of the women.

CONTRACEPTION

The traditional opposition of Catholic leaders to abortion, sterilization, and mechanical and chemical means of contraception needs no documentation here. Newer methods, such as anovulant drugs, have also been condemned: "Pius XII stated September, 1958 that a direct and therefore illicit sterilization is provoked when medicines are used to 'prevent conception by preventing ovulation.' "[26] While certain aspects are under review, the most recent statement of Pope Paul VI at the time of writing this paper reaffirmed that "chemical or mechanical means of contraception vitiate the essence of the conjugal act. Only total continence or limitation of intercourse to the infer-

[26] Cited by R. M. Fagley, "Doctrines and Attitudes of Major Religions in Regard to Fertility," Paper 92, *Proceedings of the 1965 World Population Conference* (in press).

tile female period 'on sure and sufficient moral motives' is licit, he said."[27]

With respect to attitudes we have selected two items from the questionnaire. The first reflects opinions regarding the acceptability of providing information on birth control. "Does it strike you as good or not that you be given information on birth control?" The second item taps the individual's attitude toward personal use of a relatively simple contraceptive: "There are pills to avoid getting pregnant, which are taken daily for 20 days during the month. If you could get them, would you take them?"

Rather than present the full tables, we have used index numbers in Table 29, expressing the percentage difference between the "nominals" and the "devouts" within each educational category. Thus, among better educated Bogotá women, over twice as high a proportion of "devout" as "nominal" Catholic women believe birth control information should not be distributed; and 21 percent fewer of them would take a contraceptive pill. We see that, with remarkable consistency, the more devout women have less favorable attitudes toward birth control than the nominals, while "marginal" Catholics fall in between. (The latter data are not shown in the table. In the 24 comparisons possible, "marginal" Catholics fall between the other two groups in 19 instances. In the remaining instances they "exceed" by two or three percentage points the favorable attitudes of the "nominals.") Further, on the information item, in all cities the relation is stronger among the better educated women; but on attitude toward personal use of a pill, this is true among only half of the cities.

Table 30 shows actual experience with contraception. Women from Mexico City and Bogotá have had least experience with birth control, but about six of every ten mated women in the other cities have used a method, the most frequently declared contraceptives being douche, condom, with-

[27] *New York Times,* November 27, 1965.

Table 29. Attitude toward birth control, by education and religiosity. Index numbers for devout (nominals = 100)

City	Percent who believe birth control information should *not* be distributed			Percent who would take the contraceptive pill		
	Total	Index numbers		Total	Index numbers	
		<Primary	≥Primary		<Primary	≥Primary
Bogotá	27	140	210	51	88	79
Caracas	22	122	210	44	57	73
Mexico City	31	125	190	41	60	53
Panama City	20	111	141	50	74	64
Rio de Janeiro	50	109	119	34	68	71
San José	36	179	260	53	56	67

drawal, and rhythm. The only major variations in methods occur with respect to the unusually low incidence of use of condom and withdrawal in Rio, a datum which suggests faulty interviewing.

Table 30. Percent who have ever used specified method of birth control

City	Any method[a]	Douche	Condom	Withdrawal	Rhythm
Bogotá	40	13	10	17	19
Caracas	59	25	32	23	19
Mexico City	38	15	9	7	15
Panama City	60	26	17	11	16
Rio de Janeiro	58	24	12	5	17
San José	65	17	37	24	18
San Salvador	—	16	13	11	16

[a] Includes non-Catholic women. Taken from C. A. Miró and F. Rath, "Preliminary Findings," *op. cit.*

Of greater interest for our purpose is Table 31, showing experience with the various methods according to degree of religiosity. Differences among the less educated women were minimal, and consequently we have presented differences only for

Table 31. Ever use of specified methods of birth control by "devout" women, better educated only (index numbers: percent of "nominals" who have ever used a method = 100)

City	Douche	Condom	Withdrawal	Rhythm
Bogotá	40	43	61	80
Caracas	66	78	81	135
Mexico City	50	66	66	122
Panama City	79	54	83	153
Rio de Janeiro	61	71	120	124
San José	50	43	42	133
San Salvador	144	118	96	114

the better educated women. With the exception of San Salvador, mechanical and chemical methods have been used by smaller proportions of "devout" than of "nominal" Catholics in all cities, the differences being the greatest in Bogotá. With respect to the rhythm method however, in every city but Bogotá, between a quarter and a half more "devout" than "nominal" Catholics have used the method, clear evidence of the relation of religiosity to contraceptive behavior.

FERTILITY

While levels of fertility are high in most Latin American countries and show little signs of change, there is good reason to believe that differential fertility by major social categories exists throughout the continent.[28] Within the cities surveyed in this report, major differences by education level have already been reported,[29] and can also be observed in Table 32. Thus, by whatever means it is achieved, differential fertility does exist among urban populations. Given this fact, and given the pattern of our earlier findings, we would then expect religiosity to be positively associated with fertility. Table 32 shows that by and large this is not the case. Indeed, in several instances there is a slight *negative* association, and in the case of Lima and the better educated women of San Salvador, the negative relation is substantial.

One possible explanation for a negative relation is that we have only imperfectly controlled education. The most extreme case is in Panama where among the better educated group of women, "devouts" average almost two years more education than "nominals."

[28] See Chapter 17, and R. O. Carleton "Fertility Trends, and Differentials in Latin America," *Milbank Memorial Fund Quarterly*, XLIII (October 1965).

[29] C. Miró, "Some Misconceptions Disproved," *op. cit.*

Table 32. Mean number of live births, standardized for age,[a] by education and religious practice

City	Total	Less than primary school			Primary school and over		
		Nom-inal	Mar-ginal	De-vout	Nom-inal	Mar-ginal	De-vout
Bogotá	4.07	4.16	4.36	4.53	3.53	3.85	3.85
Caracas	3.65	4.51	3.92	3.41	3.01	2.88	3.01
Lima[b]	—	447		349	354		255
Mexico City	4.21	4.92	4.41	4.67	3.68	3.99	3.48
Panama City	3.34	4.02	3.87	3.48	3.16	2.79	2.73
Rio de Janeiro	2.72	3.35	3.06	3.05	2.23	2.39	2.07
San José	3.79	4.56	4.29	4.34	3.32	3.23	3.03
San Salvador[c]	—	393		430	373		255

[a] Standardization by direct method, using total age distribution of the six cities in the CELADE series as the standard population.
[b] Median live births per 1,000 years mated.
[c] Mean live births per 1,000 years mated. Also see notes in Tables 26 and 27.

179

Such a fact cannot of course account for the positive relation of religiosity to family size norms, attitudes to contraception, or to practice of contraception, since the relation of these to education is in the opposite direction. In any event, if we cannot infer a positive relation between religiosity and fertility, the more important conclusion is the absence of a negative relation, despite the negative relation between religiosity and practice of mechanical and chemical contraception. Possibly the more devout marry later or practice contraception more consistently once they initiate family planning, matters beyond the scope of the present paper.

NON-CATHOLICS

Since so few non-Catholic women fell in the samples under discussion, we have eliminated them from our analysis thus far. However, Table 33 gives a rapid gross comparison between them and the declared Catholic women in the samples. The comparisons are made without regard to possible demographic or socioeconomic differences between Catholics and non-Catholics. It is nevertheless interesting to see that no easy generalizations about fertility-related variables can be made about Catholic versus non-Catholic women in the major cities of Latin America.

In terms of ideal family size only two cities show differences of more than 10 percent, and in actual fertility only three. In these three, non-Catholic women have had slightly fewer births. In four cities there is a difference in excess of 10 percent with respect to attitude toward the provision of birth control information, Protestants being more favorably inclined in three of the four cases; but in terms of attitude toward taking an oral contraceptive, Catholic women in all but Caracas are more favorable. In Mexico City non-Catholic women are more likely than Catholic women to have used each of the four main con-

Table 33. Selected items relating to fertility, non-Catholic mated women (index numbers: Catholic mated women = 100)

Items	Bogotá	Caracas	Mexico City	Panama City	Rio de Janeiro	San José
Median ideal family size	96	82	85	109	101	94
Mean live births	73	110	83	89	95	99
Percent believe birth control information should not be distributed	89	92	52	175	92	72
Percent would take pill	63	107	88	81	65	81
Percent ever used douche	146	56	160	96	117	153
Percent ever used rhythm	153	74	147	112	124	100
Percent ever used condom	100	69	267	112	125	84
Percent ever used withdrawal	171	48	214	73	71	96
Number of women	(21)	(64)	(77)	(127)	(252)	(78)

181

traceptive methods, but in Caracas the Catholic women were more likely to use contraception. In other cities the situation varies according to contraceptive, but in three of the six, substantially greater proportions of non-Catholic women have practiced the rhythm technique.

CONCLUSIONS

After an analysis of national fertility levels, Day concludes that "the problem seems *not* to be one of Catholic teaching in predominantly Catholic countries. The frequently voiced hope that the Church will change its position on family planning, and thereby help to solve the population problem in areas like Latin America, appears largely irrelevant."[30] Similarly, a leading Latin American demographer states that "the doctrinaire position of the Catholic Church does not constitute an obstacle for family planning. The persistence of a very high birth rate in Latin America cannot be attributed to the predominantly Catholic conditions of the population, but to the social and economic backwardness in which they live."[31] In a general sense our findings support these positions, at least for Catholic women living in the major cities of Latin America, for we found that the average woman wants between three and four children, would favor receiving birth control information, and has practiced or will practice contraception before completion of childbearing. Further, no consistent differences were found between Catholic and non-Catholic women in attitudes, contraceptive practices or fertility.

We also found that although there is variation in fertility among the different cities and within cities among different educational strata, there is no variation in the expected direction

[30] L. Day, *op. cit.*

[31] C. Miró, "Características Demográficas de América Latina," Santiago, Series A.E./C.N. CELADE, A. 12, D. 3, 4/1, 4 Rev. 1, 1963.

according to religiosity. However, the attitudes and behavior directly relevant to fertility—attitudes toward family size and contraception, and the practice of birth control—showed consistent relationships with degree of religiosity, as measured by frequency of Communion. Thus if Catholicism is having little impact on fertility, it may be partly because the average woman is not very "Catholic" by Church standards, and partly because the attitudes and practices of the less religious woman are not especially effective in the control of fertility.

What will happen as educational levels rise, and the number of priests, now relatively low, increases? Paradoxically, while the groups most affected (in attitudes and practices) by the Church's teaching are the better educated women, the better educated women are precisely those with lower fertility. This suggests that while increases in general education may eventually lower fertility, they may also bring more psychological stresses to Catholic women acutely aware of the discrepancy between the Church's position and their own needs and wishes. Lower fertility levels will be achieved at the cost of personal stress and, ultimately, of stresses on the Church. On the other hand, there is the possibility that Church teaching will move closer to present-day realities in Latin America. As Father Gustavo Perez has put it, "I share the hopes of many in Latin America who expect a public statement in Schema 13, that there is a need for Responsible Parenthood; that the Church today is not pro-natalist and does not necessarily favor large families in all circumstances."[32]

[32] G. Pérez, "Políticas de Investigación sobre Planificación de la Familia en América Latina," O.A.S. Department of Social Affairs, UP/Ser. H/VII. 39, July 1965.

III

SOCIAL AND DEMOGRAPHIC
CONTEXTS OF FERTILITY

12

Norms and Sexual
Relations in Jamaica

One of the characteristic features of reproduction in Latin America is the righ rate of illegitimacy evidenced by many countries. To a large extent this is due to frequency of *de facto* or consensual unions. While in many instances these unions are as stable as legal marriages, on the whole they are less stable. The consequences of this fact for fertility have only recently been realized.

In the English-speaking Caribbean, both illegitimacy rates and the instability of conjugal unions have been particularly high, making this area especially interesting for the study of fertility. The theory popular among many intellectuals of the region is that high rates of promiscuity produce high fertility. Lower-class sexual behavior is largely seen as instinctive and uninhibited by norms, reproduction as a generally desirable by-product of the carefree mingling of the sexes.

This idyllic view of the lower classes has only a vague resemblance to the true situation, for there are norms about sexual behavior and reproduction not so different from middle-class norms. These norms do affect behavior, and do in fact both directly and indirectly limit fertility. As we will see in the following section, the norms affect the frequency of sexual relations both within and outside of marriage, while the very instability of the unions reduces the exposure to conception.

In Chapter 9 we reported briefly the results of a national

survey on fertility in Jamaica. As part of this survey we selected for reinterview a subsample of 75 urban women of varying rates of reproduction in order better to account for differential fertility. The subsample was stratified according to the three categories of marital status and three categories of fertility (apparently sterile, infertile, and highly fertile). From each of the resulting nine strata, eight or nine cases were selected at random.

A new interviewing schedule was drawn up, largely employing qualitative interviewing techniques. The two supervisors and the two top interviewers were used to collect the data. The interview guide stressed the marital history, in an attempt to discover whether the pattern of marital relationships might be related to attitudes toward and behavior bearing on fertility. These data permit us to see most vividly the impact of the marriage norm on behavior patterns, which in turn affect fertility.

The first sexual relationship of a more or less regular nature typically occurs while the girl is living at home. Seventy-two percent of the subsample's first visiting relations occurred while the respondent was living at home, and in another 16 percent the respondent had been living with other older individuals. The parents, more often the mother or grandmother, tend to object to the relationship both because the daughter is "too young" and because they have hopes of her eventually settling into a married relationship. Therefore the suitors find great difficulty in visiting the girl at her home.

He never came home. My parents were opposed.

He couldn't come to the yard. Grandma was too strict.

He could come whenever he wanted, but just to the gate.

They wouldn't allow him at home.

How many potential relationships such restrictions curtail cannot be estimated from our present sample, in which all such unions involved sexual relations. There seems little doubt, however, that parental surveillance greatly reduced the opportunities for intercourse.

We could only have relations when he happened to find me alone at home, and that wasn't often.

We could have relations only now and again as mother was very strict.

He would come when my parents were away. We only had sex once and I got pregnant.

We only had relations twice. When he came I was not allowed to go out with him.

In the absence of parents, parental surrogates (an older sister, an aunt, or other relatives) play a similar role. Some girls who worked as maids also expressed the difficulty of meetings with men when they were required to live on the premises. Of all girls not living alone at the time of first union half said they had difficulty in seeing their boyfriends because of supervision, and another 13 percent said the affair was clandestine. Only about a third said they had no difficulty with parents or parental surrogates.

Domiciliary location is somewhat related to the frequency of visiting, but markedly related to sexual frequency, as shown in Table 34. Thus, it is probable that living with guardians created

Table 34. Median monthly frequency of sexual relations and visiting, according to residential status for all visiting relations

Residential status	Visiting	Sex relations
Lived alone	16 (41)	8 (40)
Lived with others	12 (121)	3 (118)

general obstacles to visiting, but placed *specific* obstacles in the way of sexual relations.

In addition to the watchful eyes of those responsible for the young girl, she herself, when aware of the possible consequences of sexual relationships, is often fearful of pregnancy—not, it should be noted, of pregnancy per se, but of pregnancy while in a single status. More often than not, however, the fear was expressed in terms of the reactions of the parents.

My mother was so strict that I was afraid to go to her with belly.

I couldn't think of getting pregnant as I was living in my mother's home.

I didn't want to get pregnant as I was afraid of mother.

While not explicit in most cases, a number of references make it clear that these fears may have led to actions which reduced the exposure to conception.

I just thought it wouldn't look decent for him to come often.

I know how displeased my mother would be so I asked him to lessen his visits.

I told him not to bother me for I wouldn't want to get impregnant while with my mother and father.

Such comments are to be contrasted with those in which the girl or her parents believed that the relationship would or could lead to marriage. In such instances, parental supervision was relaxed, the fear of pregnancy less salient, and sexual frequency consequently higher.

My parents approved because he said he would marry me.

I knew he would marry me so there was no holding back.

He suggested marriage so it [the visiting relation] was OK with mother.

My parents approved after he declared his intention.

[We did it often] because I thought he would marry me.

In some instances the male held out marriage as the "bait" for sexual relations, while in others the female offered herself freely in the hope that a pregnancy would induce the male to marry.

The effect of the marriage norm on sexual frequency, then, seems evident. Where marriage is the value or goal but not the expectation with regard to the first suitor, behavior of the parent or parental surrogate and of the girl herself is often such as to lessen the risk of conception by reducing the frequency of sexual contact. This appears to be the more typical pattern seen in first relationships. Where marriage is expected or viewed as realizable, both internal and external controls are relaxed. If the foregoing be true, we would expect sexual frequency to increase upon marriage. This hypothesis will be examined subsequently in more detail, but the following quotation is a rather extraordinary illustration of how sexual behavior can be regulated by a complex of expectations and goals.

I do it more often with this one than I did with H. because I feel he will marry me. But we don't have relations as often as he would like . . . as I tell him I don't want to get pregnant before marriage.

Thus the combination of an expectation of marriage but the present failure to have achieved such a status appears to have affected a compromise sexual frequency—less than would be the case if married, but more than was the case when marriage was not in sight.

THE SECOND VISITING RELATIONSHIP

The second union, even if it is a visiting relationship, shows a pattern of increased sexual frequency and regularity. One explanation for this increase lies in the fact that fewer girls are at this point living at home and more are living by themselves. Although in only 6 percent of the first visiting unions was the girl living alone, the percentage rises to 29, 48, and 70 for visiting unions of the second, third, and higher order. The absence of parental surveillance removes one obstacle to sexual relations. But even where the girl remains at home, there appears to be a relaxation of the earlier restrictions. Thus, whereas only 37 percent of those living at home during their first union said they experienced no difficulties, 60 percent reported no difficulties for subsequent visiting relations. "They liked him better" is the typical response to the question concerning parental attitudes with regard to the second union. Since the girl will often have had a child by this time, the parents may become more resigned to a visiting status, especially as the additional income provided by the partner may allay the expenses of the child. Moreover, the girl is older, may be earning money herself, and may be viewed more as an adult. As one respondent put it: "I was supporting my mother. She couldn't say anything."

Increasing age produces changes in attitude on the part of the girl as well as her parents. A number of respondents in explaining their increased sexual frequency in the second relationship mentioned their ignorance of sex in the first relation or their feeling of domination by their parents.

I was so young and green I did not want to do anything against my people.

With the first one I was very young and we had to hide. He was very young too.

With this one I was growing up, and hearing other people talk I got more the sense of everything [with reference to sex].

With the first I was green, but then I got to understand the business better as time grew.

Not only does the girl by this time have more knowledge of sex, but her increased age and experience appear to enable her to make a more successful match the second time. Considering the very early age of first unions and the restrictions placed on the girl's freedom, it may be that the choice of the first partner involves little thought on the part of the girl. When asked to explain their higher sexual frequency in the second visiting relation, the large number of responses such as "I loved him more" suggests improved selective procedures.

In any event, as indicated in Table 35, the average monthly frequency of intercourse in visiting relationships shows a substantial increase after the first union. While a similar trend appears in the case of the cohabiting couples, the difference is much smaller.

Another indication is provided by the respondent's own evaluation of relative sexual frequency. In the 31 instances in which both the first and second unions were of visiting status, two-thirds reported sexual relations to be "more frequent" in the second than in the first.

Table 35. Monthly frequency of sexual relations by partner number and type union (in percent)

Monthly frequency	First partner		Subsequent partners	
	Visiting	Cohabiting	Visiting	Cohabiting
1 or less	23	0	17	2
2	22	0	18	0
3–4	33	14	22	14
5–8	15	29	25	31
9+	7	57	18	53
Total	100	100	100	100
Mean	3.6	11.7	5.8	13
Number of unions	(60)	(21)	(87)	(64)

SEXUAL RELATIONS AND FERTILITY

The infrequency of sexual relations in the visiting union is of special interest because of the possible implications for fertility. Fortunately we need not rely entirely on the small and special sample here described. For all visiting unions of women in the sample of 1,400 the following question was asked, "How often did you have sex relations with him?" The frequency from this set of data is higher than that derived from the smaller sample. Thus, whereas only 22 percent of the first visiting relations of women in the small sample reported frequencies higher than once per week, 35 percent of those in the larger sample did so. Nevertheless, the significant point here is that even the latter figure is low compared, for example, with American rates of intercourse within marriage. For the married American female active population of ages 16–20, 21–25, and 26–30, Kinsey reports median weekly frequencies of 2.8, 2.5, and 2.2.[1] In our large sample, the median for all visiting unions is only 1.6, and for first unions 1.3. Even if we exclude those who report some absolute number of relations the proportion of first unions showing weekly frequencies of at least three amounts to only 15 percent. Thus, if Jamaican rates in marriage are comparable to American rates, the frequency of intercourse in the visiting status falls considerably short of those in marriage. Again, contrary to the known relation between age and sexual frequency, higher order visiting unions show higher frequency of intercourse, possibly reflecting the greater freedom from surveillance which comes with age. But even in fourth visiting unions, over a quarter had relations less than once a week and the median weekly frequency is only 2.2 (Table 36). Since very few women ever have a fourth visiting union, only a small proportion of women ever achieve such relatively high frequencies in a visiting relation.

Do our own data support the hypothesis of a positive relation between fertility and frequency of sexual intercourse? Not unequivocally. If we take women whose first union ended in a visiting relation or who are still in a visiting relation, we find that the mean number of live births per thousand mated years is 235

[1] A. Kinsey, W. Pomeroy, C. Martin, and P. H. Gebhard, *Sexual Behavior in the Human Female* (Philadelphia: W. B. Saunders, 1953), Table 93, p. 394.

Table 36. Frequency of sexual relations in visiting unions, by
union number—larger sample (in percent)

Frequency	Union				
	Total	1st	2nd	3rd	4th
Some absolute number	11	15	9	5	5
"Infrequently" or less					
than 1 per week	26	29	24	18	23
1 per week	21	21	22	25	17
2 per week	24	23	26	24	22
3+ per week	18	13	19	28	33
Total	100	101	100	100	100
Number of unions	(2,081)	(1,055)	(598)	(275)	(153)

for those with frequencies of less than once per week, 292 for
frequencies of once per week, 328 for frequencies of twice per
week, for those with three or more per week it drops to 254. In
our data the high rates for those with an absolute number can
easily be explained—any relationship which resulted in pregnancy was defined by us as a union, whereas ephemeral contacts
which did not result in pregnancy were not included as unions.
Moreover, a brief visiting relation which resulted in pregnancy
would surely be better remembered that one which did not. The
drop in fertility by the group with the highest frequency of
sexual relations (three or more times per week) is more difficult
to explain, but may reflect the lower sperm counts per copulation
which are found with more advanced frequencies.

On the other hand, our data on sexual frequency may not be
sufficiently precise or reliable for the computation of differential
fertility rates. Data collected in the United States under more
favorable field conditions show a definite relation between frequency of intercourse and speed of conception. In a study by
MacLeod and Gold, the percentage of couples conceiving in less
than six months time was only 17 percent for couples with
sexual frequencies of less than once per week. The percentages
rise steadily with increasing sexual frequencies, and of those who

averaged four or more times per week, the conception rate was 83 percent.[2] The authors then controlled for age of husband and reached a conclusion of considerable significance for our study:

At *any* frequency of intercourse, the age group under 25 years always produces a higher percentage of conceptions within six months than any age category above 25. The contrast is striking, particularly when one compares the age group below 25 with the 35 years and over group. But even in the 25–29 age group, the slowing up in ability to produce conception within the six-month period is quite evident. What is just as evident however, is the fact that, at any age level (with two exceptions) the proportion of conceptions achieved in less than six months rises with the frequency of intercourse. That is to say, the frequency of intercourse is a strong determining factor in ease of conception, no matter what the age of the husband (and obviously, of the wife), even though the chances of such conception diminish with increasing age." [3]

These conclusions, showing the strong and independent relation of age and sexual frequency to conception, help to explain the low fertility of our sample women: (1) Visiting relations are characterized by relatively infrequent sexual relations. (2) A high proportion of total mating experience is spent in visiting time, and this is especially true in the earlier unions of women,

[2] J. MacLeod and R. Z. Gold, "The Male Factor in Fertility and Infertility: VI. Semen Quality and Certain Other Factors in Relation to Ease of Conception," *Fertility and Sterility*, IV (1953), 10–33. In this connection, not only the relative frequency of intercourse but the absolute number of copulations is pertinent. Pearl estimated that an average of 244 potentially effective copulations take place per live birth, the figure based on a study of Baltimore white women. Eaton and Mayer, based on research with the extremely fertile Hutterite women, concluded that an average of 108 copulations take place. See J. W. Eaton and A. J. Mayer, *Man's Capacity to Reproduce* (Glencoe: Free Press, 1954), pp. 29–30. When we consider that terminated visiting relations last only a little over a year, and that average weekly frequency of intercourse is less than one, the low fertility of visiting relations seems quite reasonable.

[3] MacLeod and Gold, *op. cit.*, p. 29.

prior to age 30. (3) Therefore, fertility may be lowered both because of periods of nonexposure *between* unions (and most turnover occurs prior to age 30) and because a considerable proportion of *intraunion* time in the most fertile age period is characterized by infrequent sex relations. Furthermore, by the time the female enters a domiciliary relation, age reduces the chances for conception both by lowering fecundity and, should, according to data collected in the United States, reduce the frequency of intercourse. That this frequency in fact appears high relative to that characteristic of visiting relations shows the infrequency of coitus in the visiting status.

IRREGULARITY OF SEXUAL RELATIONS IN VISITING UNIONS

Thus far we have concentrated on the average frequency of sexual relations, but in terms of fertility regularity of these relations must also be considered. The evidence suggests that visiting relationships involve rather erratic patterns of sexual union, with frequent periods of separation on the part of the partners. This seems attributable not only to the difficulties inherent in the relationship, but also to its tenuous nature, involving little responsibility on the part of one partner to the other. Unlike marriage, or to a lesser extent common law unions, the visiting relation must depend for its stability mainly, if not exclusively, on the sexual or romantic bond between the participants. The freedom of the relation means not only that dissolution is frequent, but that temporary lapses are common throughout the duration of the union.

I haven't seen him for five months now.

When we have a fuss I don't see him. We had a little contention recently and I haven't seen him for two months now.

197

The nature of the unions is such that little explanation for absences is required. It seems more or less expected that these will occur.

I lost sight of him for nine weeks . . . I never asked him what happened.

He went away about three months recently. I just check him off, as I was fed up like, but since two months he is back.

Sometimes I don't see him . . . me never ask him why him no come and him never tell me.

Another reason for irregularity as well as low frequency of sexual relations in a visiting relationship may be that the woman is competing with other women for demands on her partner's time.

He'd disappear for two or three weeks at a time. He was wild and had had somebody else.

He wasn't too regular. He was busy with other women.

There were periods up to two weeks when I didn't see him. . . . He had plenty girl friends.

If the partner is in a more stable relationship with another woman then his major responsibilities are clear.

He was a man with a wife and naturally . . . he can't come to see me as often as I would like. . . . You can't make a man want you more than his wife if they are still having feeling for each other.

He didn't come regularly. He lived with another girl and had a baby to worry about.

More quantitative evidence stems from the 1,400 interviews. Interviewers were instructed to record any periods of absence during a marital union. Since this question was not explicitly written in on the questionnaire, the data at hand no doubt represent an underestimate. Moreover, such data are especially prone to error through faulty memory. We can reduce the latter source of error somewhat by considering only women aged 15 to 24 whose unions are relatively recent: 4 percent of those who are married, 3 percent of those in common law, but 13 percent of those in visiting relations mentioned at least one absence of their current partners in excess of three months. (The difference between the visiting and others is statistically significant. Differences at older ages are not significant.) Moreover, while the median total absence time (for all unions combined) was only six months for common law and six months for married women, the average separation period was twelve months for visiting women.

A final factor which leads to irregularity of sexual relations among visitors is the relative freedom and ease with which the woman can deny the male sexually. This is coupled with a greater reluctance to become pregnant.

I was always worried as I didn't want any children before marriage. . . . I used to ask him not to visit often as he was so loving, and I would try to avoid sex at times.

I never want to have any children. I don't tell him not to come here, but I get vexed first as soon as he comes and when I am vexed he doesn't bother me.

I asked him to stay off sometimes as I was afraid of getting pregnant then.

THE DOMICILIARY UNION—COMMON LAW AND MARRIAGE

With the difficulties in the way of frequent and regular sexual relations in the visiting relation, it is to be expected that the common law union would show an increase in frequency and regularity of sexual relations. The great discrepancy in sexual frequency between visiting and cohabiting statuses might to some extent be due to assortative mating; i.e., cohabiting relations may be an index of high sexual compatibility. That the *status* rather than the individuals concerned is the crucial determinant is clearly indicated by data on relationships in which the status changed but the partners remained constant. In such cases we asked the respondent whether her sexual frequency increased, decreased, or remained the same after changing from a visiting to a domiciliary status. The question was repeated with reference to sexual regularity. In 51 such changes, frequency increased in 46 (90 percent); and regularity increased in 35 (70 percent). By far the most frequent reason given by respondents was in terms of convenience.

He and me did live in the same room.

We didn't have to hide.

We could do as we liked.

Not only does the fact of living together make relations more convenient, but they are harder to avoid than in the visiting condition.

Even if I wanted to dodge it, it was hard to do it since we lived together.

Presumably, too, since the common law union is a public phenomenon, there is more expectation of sexual relations and pregnancy and children than in the visiting relation. These factors were rarely mentioned, however, as an explanation for increased sexual exposure in the common law union. Instead they are characteristic of *marriage*. Here, in addition to convenience, there is the explicit recognition that sexual relations within marriage are socially sanctioned.

It supposed to be since we are man and wife.

It was more convenient and we were married.

We are always with each other and we are married.

Living together that is more expected.

   The total consequence of living in a socially sanctioned relationship also relieves anxieties on the part of the female. This state of mind viewed as "contentment" or "happiness" also aids in increasing sexual frequency. The statements below were given in explanation of increased relations.

I feel better off in my mind.

I am feeling better because we decide to settle together and make life.

I'm more contented in my mind.

   The expectation of stability also relieves tensions which may have interfered with sexual relations.

Now we are making life together, is a better feeling . . . is not that any of us think that the other running away.

   Finally, it is only in the marital condition that reproduction receives full social sanction. Achievement of the marriage state not only relieves anxieties about pregnancy, but produces positive incentives to reproduction.

I didn't want many children before. . . . Now we're both anxious to have more children.

We're more regular now. I'm not afraid of getting pregnant.

. . . because we wanted a baby.

As we were married we were anxious to start a family.

   With this background on the common law union, we may move to a more general consideration of its incidence and relation to fertility.

13

Consensual Unions and Fertility

While the incidence of such marriage forms is especially high in the Caribbean, Latin American nations generally have much higher rates than most North American or European nations. Thus, in 1950, of twenty Latin American nations, seven recorded over 40 percent of all current unions as consensual.[1] Whether there is a relation between fertility and consensual unions in Latin America is unknown. The present paper opens up the question by using a comparison of Puerto Rico and Jamaica as a point of departure.

A comparison of Puerto Rico and Jamaica should be especially instructive, since the islands, despite having much in common geographically, historically, and economically, have evidenced highly divergent fertility patterns. As an example, in the period 1945–1949 their crude birth rates averaged 40.8 and 31.3 respectively, while in 1962 the differences were reversed—Puerto Rico's rate having dropped to 31.7, while Jamaica's increased to 42.7. The former set of figures had probably been stable for some time, and our comparative analysis of the fertility of the two islands will concentrate on the earlier situation. Both the Jamaican census of 1943 and the Puerto Rican census of 1950

[1] If we assume that Argentina and Uruguay, where data are lacking, have less than a fifth of their mated women in consensual unions, then a third of the Latin American nations show rates under 20 percent, a third from 20 to 39 percent, and a third 40 percent and higher. Computed from data in Giorgio Mortara, *Características de Estructura Demográfica de los Países Americanos* (Washington, D.C.: Instituto Interamericano de Estadística, 1961), Table IV, 2a–b, pp. 92–93.

provide us with an excellent measure of fertility—cumulative
number of live births borne by women of specified ages.

From Table 37 it is clear that Puerto Rican women in 1950
were much more prolific than Jamaican women, the difference

Table 37. Various measures of fertility, by age, Puerto Rico (1950)
and Jamaica (1943)

Age	Children per woman		Percent fertile[a]		Children per mother	
	Puerto Rico	Jamaica	Puerto Rico	Jamaica	Puerto Rico	Jamaica
15–19	0.2	0.2	25	13	1.5	1.3
20–24	1.4	1.0	57	48	2.4	2.0
25–29	2.7	1.9	78	64	3.5	3.0
30–34	3.8	2.8	85	72	4.5	3.9
35–44	5.1	3.9	87	79	5.8	5.0
45–54	5.6	4.8	86	83	6.5	5.7
55–64	5.7	5.0	87	84	6.8	6.0

[a] At least one child ever born.

Sources: *1943 Census of Jamaica*, Table 40, p. 57; *1950 U.S. Census of Population, Puerto Rico*, P-c53, Table 51, pp. 53–120.

ranging between 30 and 40 percent for the various five-year age
groups. Although by the end of the childbearing period almost
as high a proportion of Jamaican as Puerto Rican women have
ever borne a child, Puerto Rican women begin much earlier.
Moreover, at every age, there are still substantial differentials
when only women of proven fertility ("mothers") are compared.

Some explanation for this finding is contained in Table 38
which shows that in the earlier age groups twice as high a
proportion of Puerto Rican as Jamaican women are currently
mated (i.e., living in a married or consensual state), and even for
the ages 45–59, the difference is substantial. However, the differences in proportions mated account for only a small proportion
of Puerto Rico's higher fertility; for when only *currently mated*

Table 38. Marital status, by age, Puerto Rico (1950) and Jamaica (1943) (in percent)

	15–19		20–24		25–29		30–34		35–39		40–44		45–49	
	Puerto Rico	Ja-maica	Puerto Rico	Ja-maica	Puerto Rico	Ja-maica	Puerto Rico	Ja-maica	Puerto Rico	Ja-maica	Puerto Rico	Ja-maica	Puerto Rico	Ja-maica
Married	12.4	1.7	44.2	10.6	59.9	23.3	62.7	33.2	61.6	38.9	59.1	42.4	57.8	43.8
Common law	6.3	5.3	16.8	23.6	19.7	29.8	21.0	28.1	21.8	24.7	19.0	18.8	15.6	13.6
Total	18.7	7.0	61.0	34.2	79.6	53.1	83.7	61.3	83.4	63.6	78.1	61.2	73.4	57.4

Sources: 1943 Census of Jamaica, Table 36, p. 55; 1950 U.S. Census, Puerto Rico, Table 46, pp. 53–112.

women are considered (as contrasted with all women in Table 37), fertility differences between Puerto Rico and Jamaica are still substantial prior to age 45 (Table 39).

Table 39. Children ever born, by age, for cohabiting women (married and common law), Puerto Rico (1950) and Jamaica (1943)

Age	Children per woman		Percent fertile[a]		Children per mother	
	Puerto Rico	Jamaica	Puerto Rico	Jamaica	Puerto Rico	Jamaica
15–19	0.9	0.8	58	52	1.5	1.4
20–24	2.1	1.6	84	70	2.4	2.3
25–29	3.2	2.5	91	77	3.5	3.3
30–34	4.2	3.4	92	82	4.6	4.2
35–44	5.5	4.6	92	86	5.9	5.4
45–54	6.0	5.5	91	87	6.6	6.3
55–64	6.3	6.0	92	90	6.9	6.6

[a] At least one child ever born.
Sources: 1943 Census of Jamaica, Table 40, p. 57; *1950 U.S. Census of Population, Puerto Rico*, P-c53, Table 51, pp. 53–120.

Of mated couples, the proportion in consensual unions is twice as high in Jamaica as in Puerto Rico among women under 35, and higher at all ages under 50 (Table 40). Tables 41 and 42

Table 40. Percent common law of currently cohabiting females, by age, Puerto Rico (1950) and Jamaica (1943)

Age	Puerto Rico	Jamaica
15–19	34	76
20–24	28	69
25–29	25	56
30–34	25	46
35–39	26	39
40–44	24	31
45–49	21	24
50–54	19	16
55–59	16	12

Sources: 1943 Census of Jamaica, Table 37, p. 55; *1950 U.S. Census of Population, Puerto Rico*, Table 46, pp. 53–112.

Table 41. Children ever born to common law women, by age,
Puerto Rico (1950) and Jamaica (1943)

Age	Births per common law woman		Percent mothers		Births per common law mother	
	Puerto Rico	Jamaica	Puerto Rico	Jamaica	Puerto Rico	Jamaica
15–19	0.9	0.7	60	50	1.5	1.4
20–24	2.3	1.5	87	67	2.6	2.3
25–29	3.6	2.4	92	76	4.0	3.2
30–34	4.6	3.2	92	80	5.0	4.0
35–44	5.5	4.2	91	83	6.0	5.0
45 +	5.7	4.8	89	85	6.4	5.6

Sources: See Table 39.

consider separately the fertility of women living in legal and those living in consensual relations. From these tables we find that the major share of the remaining differential fertility occurs among consensually married rather than legally married women. Indeed, when births per married mother are considered, the difference between Jamaica and Puerto Rico virtually disappears.

Table 42. Children born to married women, by age,
Puerto Rico (1950) and Jamaica (1943)

Age	Births per married woman		Percent mothers		Births per married mother	
	Puerto Rico	Jamaica	Puerto Rico	Jamaica	Puerto Rico	Jamaica
15–19	0.9	0.8	58	60	1.5	1.4
20–24	2.0	1.8	84	74	2.4	2.4
25–29	3.1	2.7	91	79	3.4	3.4
30–34	4.2	3.6	92	83	4.5	4.4
35–44	5.6	4.9	92	87	6.1	5.6
45 +	6.6	5.9	92	89	7.2	6.6

Sources: See Table 39.

In the case of consensually mated woman, differences are substantial both in proportions who are mothers and in the fertility of mothers.

But the assumption that fertility is confined to consensually and legally married women is unwarranted. In Jamaica, the proportion of *single* women who report at least one birth rises from half the women 25–29, to two-thirds of those 35–44, and 70 percent of those over 45. In Puerto Rico the corresponding proportions are only 17, 34, and 36 percent (Table 43).

Table 43. Children born to currently single women, by age, Puerto Rico (1950) and Jamaica (1943)

Age	Births per single woman		Percent mothers		Births per mother	
	Puerto Rico	Jamaica	Puerto Rico	Jamaica	Puerto Rico	Jamaica
15–19	0.2	0.1	1	10	1.6	1.2
20–24	0.2	0.6	8	37	2.1	1.8
25–29	0.5	1.2	17	48	2.7	2.5
30–34	0.9	1.7	26	56	3.3	3.1
35–44	1.4	2.5	34	65	4.2	3.9
45+	1.9	3.3	36	70	5.2	4.7

Sources: See Table 39.

The fertility data discussed thus far are summarized in Table 44. The comparative fertility advantage of Puerto Rico is seen to be composed of very different elements—lower fertility of single women, slightly higher fertility of married women, and much higher fertility of consensually married women.

The higher fertility of Jamaican currently single women is due to the fact that more of them have had a child. The fertility of single *mothers* is only slightly less than in Puerto Rico—the differences less than 10 percent in most age groups. While the fertility of Jamaican single women is high relative to the Puerto

Table 44. Comparison between Puerto Rico and Jamaica in births per woman, by age and marital status (index numbers: Jamaica = 100)

Age	All women	Currently mated	Con-sensual	Married	Single
20–24	140	131	153	111	25
25–29	142	128	150	115	37
30–34	136	124	144	117	51
35–44	131	120	131	114	58
45+	—	—	119	112	57

Rican single, it is low compared to the fertility of the concensually or legally married in either place. Thus, the net effect of the high proportion of single women in Jamaica is to lower overall fertility relative to Puerto Rico.

But why are common law unions so much more fertile in Puerto Rico than in Jamaica? Our hypothesis is that the Puerto Rican consensual union is much more stable than the Jamaican. Unlike broken marriages, which are classified as widowed, divorced or separated, broken consensual unions are not recorded at all. Many Jamaican women recorded as "single" had past consensual unions; whereas we believe that this is much less true for Puerto Rico.

We saw from Table 38 that for age groups over 30, about 40 percent of Jamaican women but only about 20 percent of Puerto Rican women were single; on the other hand, as seen in Table 43, most of the single Jamaican women have had a child, while most of the Puerto Rican women have not. The differential incidence of single women compared with the differential fertility of single women in the two islands may reflect differences in the stability of consensual unions in Puerto Rico and Jamaica.[2]

While the data suggest that consensual unions reduce fertility in Jamaica, such unions apparently have no such impact in Puerto

[2] A sample census of Jamaica in 1953 indicated that the mean length of current union for common law women aged 45 and over was only 15.2 years (as opposed to 20.8 years for married women).

Rico, where at ages prior to 35, they show *higher* fertility than married unions. However, the consensual union is a minority mating pattern in Puerto Rico, while in Jamaica the majority of mated females are in such unions prior to age 30 (Table 39). In Puerto Rico, therefore, it may be confined to the poorest and least educated classes in society. Such characteristics should be held constant in comparing fertility in varying marital statuses, and it is possible to do so for 1960 Puerto Rican census data. For this reason, and because the Puerto Rican experience may be more relevant than the Jamaican for Latin American countries, we turn to a more detailed examination of the consensual union in Puerto Rico.

At the turn of the century, about one out of every three mated Puerto Rican women was reported by the census as living in a consensual union. The two decades following American occupation of Puerto Rico brought a sharp decline to a proportion of one in four, a level that was maintained between 1920 and 1940. Between 1940 and 1960, and coinciding with the decades of Puerto Rico's economic take-off, another decline is evident, accelerated between 1950 and 1960. In the latter year, only 14.3 percent of the mated females and 13.5 percent of the mated males were reported as consensual. Between 1940 and 1950 the decline was largely among younger couples, but by 1960 every age group registered marked declines from the earlier decade.

An unusual opportunity for examining the relation between fertility and consensual unions is afforded by special tabulations of the 1960 census. Tabulated by the Puerto Rican Planning Board for the International Population Program, the data are based on the 25 percent sample of ever-married and consensually married women. The measure of fertility used is the mean number of children ever born alive per 1,000 women. To eliminate the effects of differential age distributions among the categories compared, a direct standardization technique was employed, using the age distribution of the total sample as the standard population.

As seen in Table 45, a positive relation between fertility and consensual unions is again apparent in 1960, the age-standardized

Table 45. Births per 1,000 "ever-married" women by age and marital status, Puerto Rico, 1960

Age	Intact unions		Broken unions
	Married	Con-sensual	(Widowed-divorced-separated)
15–19	1,007	1,289	1,625
20–24	2,129	2,881	2,174
25–29	3,118	4,305	3,042
30–34	4,031	5,415	3,877
35–44	5,346	6,437	4,799
45+	6,222	6,021	6,151
Total	4,564	5,003	4,706
Age-standardized total[a]	4,723	5,309	4,210

[a] Standardized by the direct method, using the age distribution of all women 15 and over reporting on fertility.

number of live births 12 percent higher for the consensual than for the married women. With increasing age, however, the fertility differentials by marital status tend to decrease. In the age groups 20–34, consensually mated women show over a third more births than married women; in the age group 35–44 the differential drops to about a fifth; and for women 45 and over the relation disappears or goes slightly in the opposite direction. In Table 46 fertility is further broken down into two components —proportions infertile and the level of fertility of mothers. While the latter pattern is little different from that shown in Table 45, the proportions childless reflect the pattern in a more dramatic fashion. Whereas at ages 20–24 there are twice as many childless among the married as among the consensual, by age 35 the consensual women show higher proportions of childless than the married. A possible explanation of this surprising relation is that consensually married women who have no children or few

Table 46. Fertility measures by age and marital status of women,
Puerto Rico, 1960

Age	Number of childless per 1,000 women			Births per 1,000 mothers		
	Married	Consensual	Wid., Div., and Sep.	Married	Consensual	Wid., Div., and Sep.
15–19	378	326	305	1,618	1,912	1,625
20–24	148	72	123	2,500	3,103	2,174
25–29	71	44	66	3,355	4,502	3,042
30–34	52	48	57	4,250	5,687	3,877
35–44	53	60	66	5,647	6,850	4,799
45+	83	98	80	6,787	6,673	6,151
Total	89	85	85	5,008	5,470	5,147
Age-standard-ized total[a]	90	82	86	5,180	5,823	4,616

[a] Births per mother standardized by the direct method, utilizing the age distribution of all reporting mothers.
Source: Special tabulations, 1960 Census.

children may be *less likely to legitimatize their union*.[3] We have already seen that the consensual unions decline markedly with age. It is reasonable to assume that fertile women would have much more motivation to legalize their unions than the relatively infertile. On the other hand, at early ages, many consensual unions may have been precipitated by a pregnancy. Over time those unions which remain intact and are more fertile are those which are then more likely to be legitimized.

However, another explanation is also possible. Women who are still in consensual unions after age 45 are more likely to be poorly educated and rural. Of mated females aged 25–44, for example, 28 percent of those with no education, 14 percent of

[3] For a parallel phenomenon in Jamaica, see J. M. Stycos and K. W. Back, *The Control of Human Fertility in Jamaica* (Ithaca: Cornell University Press, 1965).

those with five to seven years of education, and only 7 percent of those with eight years were living in consensual unions in 1960. The apparent drops in consensual fertility occurring between ages 35–44 and 45 and over, may be due to an underreporting tendency on the part of these women. Thus the drop does *not* occur in the San Juan metropolitan area, where we would most expect it to if the hypothesis of legitimization just advanced were true.

In Table 47, the age-standardized totals suggest that the higher fertility of consensual unions is largely an *urban* phenomenon;[4] however, examination of the data by age group shows that in the

Table 47. Births per thousand women by marital status, residence, and labor force status of female (age standardized), Puerto Rico, 1960

Labor force status	Married	Con- sensual	Wid., div., sep.	Total
Rural				
In labor force	4,492	5,066	4,039	4,385
Not in labor force	5,879	5,852	5,168	5,728
Total	5,703	5,776	4,976	5,550
Urban				
In labor force	2,946	3,734	2,996	3,010
Not in labor force	4,282	4,771	4,138	4,300
Total	3,970	4,604	3,797	3,984
San Juan				
In labor force	2,529	4,129	2,690	2,669
Not in labor force	3,983	5,005	4,002	4,109
Total	3,668	4,860	3,583	3,766
Total				
In labor force	3,282	4,412	3,142	3,296
Not in labor force	5,030	5,439	4,575	4,965
Total	4,723	5,309	4,210	4,648

Source: Special tabulations, 1960 Census.

[4] This was also true in 1950, the married-consensual differential greater in urban than in rural areas at all ages. From age 35 on in rural areas, legally married women show more births per woman than did the consensually married.

rural area, superior consensual fertility is characteristic of every age group up to 45. The size of the older age group is such that it pulls the mean close to its value.

The greatest differences occur among the groups of highest status. For example, there is no difference in fertility by marital status among rural women not in the labor force. Similarly, among those with less than five years of education, consensual unions are slightly less fertile than legal unions; while among better educated classes the consensual fertility is higher (not shown). In short, the more modern or cosmopolitan the category—urban, better educated, employed—the greater the superiority of consensual fertility. In addition to possible differential response errors, one explanation might be that urban women in consensual unions are more likely to be migrants from rural areas than are married urban women. Their fertility, therefore, might be expected to be between urban and rural levels. It might also be the case that of the rural consensual women, those with low fertility are more likely to migrate. However, as shown in an article by Myers and Morris,[5] when only *non*migrants are considered (as defined either by place of birth or place of residence five years ago), the superiority of consensual fertility is still apparent in the urban area, and not in the rural. Moreover, the fertility of the migrants is slightly lower than that of the residents. There may also be essential differences in stability of consensual unions among different classes, or the degree to which consensual unions are legitimized later in life, but data on these aspects are not available.

SUMMARY

In examining the question of a relation between consensual unions and fertility in Latin America, we examined census data from two Caribbean islands with different cultural orientations.

[5] George Myers and Earl Morris, "Migration and Fertility in Puerto Rico," *Population Studies,* XX (July 1966).

Puerto Rican women were found to be much more prolific than Jamaican, beginning reproduction earlier and continuing reproduction at higher rates. However, the varying statuses show different relationships to fertility. Thus the fertility of single Jamaican women is higher than that of single Puerto Ricans, the fertility of married Jamaicans is only slightly lower, while the fertility of the consensually married is much lower. It is probably that the common law union in Jamaica is less stable than in Puerto Rico. The high incidence of single and consensually mated women in Jamaica largely accounts for the lower rates of birth.

Unlike Jamaica, in Puerto Rico women in consensual unions show higher fertility than married women, the relationship decreasing with age. Consensual unions may be the result of accidental pregnancies more frequently than are marriages, but in time the more fertile unions may be legalized, blurring the difference in fertility between legally married women and others. On the other hand, the fertility differentials by marital status are especially marked among the urban, working and better educated women, precisely the groups for which we would expect the greater tendency toward legalization of consensual union.

14

Culture and Differential
Fertility in Peru

This chapter analyzes regional data on human fertility from
the 1940 Census of Peru. The reasons for dealing with information collected over two decades ago are several. First, scholars
have never exploited these data. Second, since no other census
was taken until 1961, the imminent availability of both new
census data and a sample survey of fertility conducted in 1961
enhances the importance of the 1940 information for comparative purposes. Third, and of immediate concern, is to determine
whether or not fertility differentials in Peru were apparent as
early as 1940, and, if so, to discover which social characteristics
were related to such differentials.

The 1940 Census of Peru presented a considerable number of
breakdowns for the 23 departments, and a lesser number of
breakdowns for the 120 provinces. The present analysis required initially the computation of a variety of social and demographic characteristics for each province and department. The
only fertility measure available for provinces was the child-
woman ratio, and, because of the system of age grouping used in
the Peruvian census, the ratio was computed as number of children under six years of age per 100 women, aged 20-59.

This crude measure shows considerable regional variation.
Lima's ratio is exceeded by 39 percent by the rest of the nation.
For the 22 departments,[1] the range is 67 to 113, with a median

[1] One department with only 813 mated women recorded has been
excluded from the present analysis (Madre de Dios).

value of 84. The metropolitan departments of Lima and Callao show the lowest ratios, 67 each. The child-woman ratio, especially the one here used, has special limitations which have caused some analysts to raise doubts about the rural-urban fertility differentials evident in many Latin American cities when this measure is employed.[2] Fortunately, more direct indices of fertility are available for the 23 departments. Table 48 presents three measures computed for Lima-Callao and the remainder of the country.

Table 48. Fertility by age and residence, Peru, 1940

Age	Live births per 100 women		Live births per 100 mothers		Percentage fertile	
	Lima-Callao	Other	Lima-Callao	Other	Lima-Callao	Other
15–19	14	13	138	136	10	9
20–24	94	108	205	202	46	54
25–29	197	240	304	316	65	76
30–34	297	368	407	433	73	85
35–39	391	475	511	542	76	88
40–44	454	545	586	614	77	89
45+	485	553	650	659	75	84

From age 25 on, each age category of women in the non-metropolitan area shows from a fifth to a quarter higher fertility than in Lima and Callao, as judged by births per 100 women. (For women aged 50 and over the difference drops to 12 percent, perhaps suggesting that differential fertility may have been less among the older generation.) Thus, although rural-urban differences were not so marked in 1940 as suggested by the child-woman ratio, they were substantial when measured by more direct means.

[2] See, e.g., W. C. Robinson and E. H. Robinson, "Rural-Urban Fertility Differentials in Mexico," *American Sociological Review*, XXV, No. I, 77–81.

When only *fertile* women are considered, however (i.e., those who have ever had a live birth), the residential differences virtually disappear, the maximum differences being of the order of only 6 percent. This suggests that differential fertility may to a large extent have been due to a higher proportion of urban women remaining childless. This is borne out by the data in the last two columns of Table 48, where substantial differences in proportions fertile appear from age 20 and continue throughout the reproductive period.

Of the departments of Peru, Lima-Callao had the next to lowest proportion of mothers aged 45 and over (75 percent; eleven provinces had 85 percent or more in this category), and the next to lowest number of live births per 100 women 45 and over. However, Lima and Callao fell exactly in the middle of the provincial distribution for numbers of live births per 100 *mothers* 45 and over. Further, only 53 percent of all Lima-Callao women aged 15 and over have ever had a child, whereas the unweighted mean percentage for the remaining departments is 68 percent.

Of the various factors which might cause a higher rate of childlessness in the metropolitan region, we have a certain amount of data on two—the incidence of marriage and age at marriage. In proportions of women aged 15 and over currently mated (legally or consensually),[3] the departments range from 41 percent to 61 percent with a median value of 52. Lima ranks sixth from the bottom with 48 percent mated. Thus the total incidence of marital unions in the city is low, but by no means the lowest in the nation.

While we lack information on age at entry to consensual unions, we do have information on age at legal marriage for recent years (see Table 49). Peruvian women in 1957 married considerably later than American women or women in our most

---

[3] Of mated women the average department had 35 percent in consensual unions, with a range from 10 to 61 percent. Thirty percent of Lima's couples were living in consensual unions in 1940.

Table 49. Age at marriage, 1958[a]

Age	Rhode Island percent	U.S.A. percent	Peru percent	Lima percent
−24	86	81	62	53
25–29	7	11	18	24
30+	7	8	20	23
Total	100	100	100	100

[a] First marriages for U.S. data. National Peruvian data for 1957. Lima data computed from *Boletín Estadístico Municipal, Ciudad de Lima, año* XXVII, No. 105–08.

Catholic and most urbanized state, Rhode Island. Whereas half of the American women who married for the first time in 1958 were under 20, just under half who married in Lima were 25 years of age or older. Just under a quarter were 30 years of age or more, an age by which most American women have already had their last child. Whether for biological or volitional reasons, it is probable that a high proportion of the marriages contracted at higher ages remain childless, unless, of course, they represent merely the legal consolidation of consensual unions contracted earlier. While this question cannot be answered at this time, there is evidence suggesting that the average Lima mother is relatively old at the birth of her first child, though not so old as the age at marriage data would indicate. The mean and median age of mothers at birth of first child for Lima in 1959 were 22.3 and 22.0.[4] Few countries in the hemisphere publish birth order data by age of mother, but Table 50 shows the low age in Lima as compared with most other *countries* for which information is available.

Lima, then, is quite distinct from the rest of Peru in terms of the proportion of women who are mothers, the age at marriage,

[4] As might be expected, illegitimate births occur earlier than legitimate. Only 24 percent of legitimate, but 41 percent of illegitimate first births occurred to Lima women under age 20 in 1959. Forty-five percent of all Lima births in 1959 were illegitimate.

Table 50. Age of mother at birth of first child (in percent)

Place and year	Age			Total
	−19	20–24	25+	
Lima, 1958–59	29	41	30	100
Chile, 1956	29	37	34	100
Puerto Rico, 1957	42	40	18	100
Guatemala, 1958	49	32	19	100
Panama, 1958	53	33	14	100
Trinidad, 1957	54	31	15	100
U.S.A., 1957	34	43	23	100

Source: Lima: special tabulations by S.C.I.S.P. Other countries: United Nations *Demographic Yearbook,* 1959.

and probably in the age of birth of first child. What of the other departments of Peru?

For each department the proportions of women who have ever borne a child, number of births per 100 women, and number of births per 100 mothers were computed for all women aged 15 and over, and again for women aged 45 and over. The Pearsonian correlations between data for women aged 15 and over and those aged 45 and over were 0.70, 0.76, and 0.94 respectively for the three measures. In each instance, the correlation between these measures and the child-woman ratio was a few points higher for women aged 45 and over than for women aged 15 and over. The interrelation of the four measures of fertility is an interesting one and is presented in Table 51. For simplicity we have used the data for women aged 45 and over. (A complete matrix of intercorrelations is presented in Table 60 of the Appendix to this chapter.) First of all, it is of interest that the child-woman ratio, for all its defects, shows a fairly close relation to births per 100 women, and only a somewhat lower relation to births per mother. Second, despite a close relation between births per woman and births per mother, and despite a positive correlation between the incidence of mother-

Table 51. Intercorrelations of fertility measures,
22 departments of Peru, 1940

Fertility measures	Child-woman ratio	Births per 100 women aged 45 and over	Births per 100 mothers aged 45 and over
Births per 100 women aged 45 and over	0.70		
Births per 100 mothers aged 45 and over	0.61	0.90	
Percentage women aged 45 and over who are mothers	0.44	0.53	0.13

hood and births per woman, there is virtually no relation between the incidence of motherhood and births per mother. This may suggest again at least two important and unrelated components making up an overall fertility rate: the proportion of women who bear at least one child, and the fertility of women once they become mothers.

Let us now look at the relation of fertility variables to three social measures—the percentage of adults literate, percentage of the department's population residing in urban places by the census definition, and percentage of the population speaking Spanish only, as opposed to an Indian language. The mean value of the three intercorrelations of these characteristics is 0.75. A consistent pattern emerges in Table 52: the social measures show a weak *positive* relation to births per women, a stronger positive relation to births per mother, and a *negative* relation to the incidence of motherhood.

It will be recalled that in comparing Lima with the rest of the country, the higher fertility of the latter was mainly accounted for by a higher incidence of mothers. Using data for all the departments confirms the negative relation between urbanization-

Table 52. Correlations between fertility measures and social
characteristics, 22 departments of Peru, 1940

Fertility measures	Per-centage urban	Per-centage literate	Per-centage Spanish-speaking
Percentage mothers aged 15 and over	–0.61	–0.53	–0.26
Percentage mothers aged 45 and over	–0.49	–0.44	–0.27
Births per 100 women aged 15 and over	–0.32	–0.20	0.08
Births per 100 women aged 45 and over	0.02	0.21	0.40
Births per 100 mothers aged 15 and over	0.17	0.29	0.48
Births per mother aged 45 and over	0.26	0.47	0.61

literacy and motherhood for the total population, but shows, especially for the Spanish-speaking variable, that the fertility of mothers is actually higher in higher-status areas.[5]

In a factor analysis of the twelve measures computed for the 22 departments, the rotated matrix shown in Appendix Table 61 gives further evidence that "fertility" is a complex of variables. The first factor can be labeled as a general fertility factor with which the incidence of motherhood shows only a moderate loading and with which the urbanism and literacy variables show virtually no relation. Spanish-speaking, however, shows a moderate loading. The second factor may be termed "socioeco-

[5] In the ten departments which may be considered Indian (less than 50 percent Spanish-speaking), the unweighted mean births per 100 mothers aged 45 and over are only 635; for the twelve departments in which a higher proportion speak Spanish, the figure is 722. Medians are 641 and 701 respectively. Within Indian areas the correlation between motherhood and motherhood fertility is − 0.15, within Spanish departments + 0.39.

nomic," with which the incidence of motherhood shows a fairly high *negative* loading, while the other fertility variables have fairly low loadings. Moreover, while the child-woman ratio and children per hundred women aged 15 and over show low negative loadings, children per mother shows low *positive* loadings. The socioeconomic variables make virtually no contribution to factors 3 and 4, other than a very small positive relation between Spanish-speaking and factor 4.

Thus our various techniques have led to similar conclusions: that the relation between social variables and general fertility is obscured by differing relations to two components of fertility— a negative relation to the incidence of motherhood and a positive relation to motherhood fertility. Further, the incidence of motherhood is best predicted by the degree of urbanization, but the degree of motherhood fertility is best predicted by ethnic group.

Let us now look more closely at these two measures, ethnic status and urbanization, examining our fertility data by age category, since the ratios used thus far refer only to women aged 15 and over, or 45 and over. In Table 53, we have chosen for comparison the five departments with less than 3 percent of the population Spanish-speaking only and the six departments with 93 percent or more. The previous low negative correlation between motherhood and Spanish-speaking was the result of the relation after age 30. Prior to this age the Indian departments show a considerably lower incidence of motherhood. After this age the Spanish-speaking departments show a lower incidence of mothers, but the difference is very small.[6]

With respect to the fertility of *mothers*, each age group shows substantially fewer births in Indian-speaking departments. After age 24, mothers in the Indian areas have about 20 percent fewer births in each age category.

---

[6] Overall higher motherhood in Indian areas is the result of differential age distribution. Probably as a result of the out-migration of young women from Indian rural areas, 32 percent of all women aged 15 and over are aged 45 and over in the most Indian areas, as opposed to only 24 percent in the most Spanish-speaking departments.

Table 53. Percentage who are mothers, and mean
births per mother by age for five departments
with smallest proportions speaking Spanish
(index numbers: six departments with highest
Spanish-speaking = 100)

Age	Percentage who are mothers	Children per mother
15–19	53	99
20–24	80	86
25–29	95	82
30–34	101	82
35–39	102	79
40–44	104	80
45–49	105	82
50 and over	102	82

If we use urbanization as our measure rather than Spanish-speaking, and compare the six departments with less than 18 percent urban population with the five departments having over 48 percent urban, the rural areas evidence 9 percent to 14 percent more mothers in each age category, but from 4 percent to 7 percent fewer births per mother than in the most urban places. Thus, as we saw earlier from the correlations in Table 52, Spanish-speaking is a better predictor of the fertility of mothers than is urbanization, but the reverse is true for the incidence of motherhood.

It would be desirable now to separate the urban variable from the cultural one (Spanish-speaking). Given the distribution of the 22 departments we can distinguish three types of departments:

(1) Those low in urban proportions (unweighted mean = 19 percent) and low in Spanish-speakers (U.M. = 7 percent).

(2) Those low in urban proportions (U.M. = 24 percent), but high in Spanish speakers (U.M. = 80 percent).

(3) Those high in urban proportions (U.M. = 57 percent) and high in Spanish speakers (U.M. = 81 percent).

In the more rural areas, the Spanish-speaking departments show a higher incidence of motherhood in almost every age category, but after age 30 the differences are trivial (Table 54). For mothers, rural Spanish areas show from 10 to 15 percent more births than rural Indian areas. Urban Spanish areas show the highest fertility of all for mothers, but the lowest incidence of motherhood after age 24. It would appear that urban residence tends to decrease motherhood and increase births per mother, but that "Spanish culture" tends to increase both. The

Table 54. Percentage who are mothers and births per mother by age and social characteristics (unweighted means)

Social characteristics	No.	Percentage who are mothers							
		15–19	20–24	25–29	30–34	35–39	40–44	45–49	50+
Rural-Indian	(8)	9	50	75	85	88	89	89	84
Rural-Spanish	(6)	14	59	80	86	89	90	91	82
Urban-Spanish	(8)	13	54	72	81	84	84	84	80
		Births per 100 mothers							
Rural-Indian	(8)	135	191	295	408	506	578	620	639
Rural-Spanish	(6)	135	210	339	464	585	652	685	681
Urban-Spanish	(8)	140	220	346	476	605	681	723	712

net effect on fertility, as measured by births per *woman* is to place the lowest fertility in the rural Indian areas, the highest fertility in the rural Spanish departments, the urban Spanish places falling in between. (See Appendix Table 58) To check this finding we can move to provincial data. Unfortunately, the only fertility measure available for provinces is the child-woman ratio. However, we saw from Table 51 that the correlation with other fertility measures is quite high. (Appendix Table 59 gives further confirmation of this fact.)

Table 55 indicates that each variable works in a different direction, Spanish-speaking provinces evidencing higher fertility in each residence class, urban provinces showing higher fertility within each cultural class. The highest fertility is again found in rural Spanish departments, the lowest in *urban* Indian departments (no such category was used in Table 54).

Table 55. Child-woman ratios for 117 provinces, by percentage speaking Spanish only and residence (unweighted means)

Percentage urban	Under half speak Spanish	Half or more speak Spanish
−14	86 (25)[a]	100 (13)
15–37	86 (31)	95 (16)
38+	84 (8)	91 (24)

[a] Figures in parentheses represent number of provinces in each cell.

The negative relation of urbanization and fertility was not unexpected, but the persistent positive relation between fertility and Spanish-speaking is surprising and may be due to some major difference between Indian and mestizo cultures in patterns of mating. Proportions married by age can unfortunately not be calculated for Peru's departments, the only available measure being proportions of all women aged 15 and over currently mated (married and common law). Although this measure shows a fairly high correlation with the child-woman ratio (0.51) and with the fertility of mothers aged 15 and over (0.50), it shows a low relation to motherhood (0.14). Correlations with the social variables are both small and in different directions: −0.14 with urbanization, −0.02 with literacy, and 0.08 with Spanish-speaking. Indeed, in the five departments with less than 3 percent Spanish-speaking and in the six with 93 percent or more Spanish-speaking (Table 53), the unweighted means for proportions mated are identical—53 percent.

Using provincial data, we find a small positive relation between proportions mated and proportions speaking Spanish, but this does not account for fertility differentials. As seen in Table 56, both Spanish-speaking and proportions mated are positively related to the child-woman ratio.

Table 56. Child-woman ratios by percentage speaking Spanish only and percentage of women aged 15 and over currently mated (unweighted means for 117 provinces)

Percent	Less than half Spanish	Half or more Spanish
Under 50 percent mated	82 (21)	89 (21)
51 percent or more mated	88 (43)	98 (32)

The finding that "marital" fertility in Indian areas is persistently lower than in Spanish-speaking areas will not surprise those who believe that altitude has a depressing effect on fertility. The belief is common, especially among those in the medical profession in Latin America, that high altitude inhibits fertility. In the present instance, there is a correlation of −0.39 between the child-woman ratio in the 117 provinces analyzed and the altitude of the provincial capitals. However, the correlation drops to −0.18 within areas with more than 50 percent Spanish-speaking (not significant at the 0.05 level) and to −0.27 within those with less than 50 percent Spanish-speaking (significant at 0.05). In Table 57, where altitude and ethnic composition are dichotomized, a small relation to fertility appears.

Unfortunately, the low-altitude Indian cell is almost empty of

Table 57. Unweighted mean child-woman ratios, by percentage Spanish-speaking and altitude, 117 provinces

Altitude	Less than half Spanish-speaking	Half or more Spanish-speaking
Under 2000 metres	94 (4)	96 (31)
2000 metres or higher	86 (60)	92 (22)

cases, and *t*-tests for the differences between the mean in this cell and the others show no significance. Among the Spanish-speaking areas the differences in fertility by altitude are not significant, but the difference between Indian and Spanish high-altitude areas by ethnic status is significant at 0.05. In short, at least as measured by the child-woman ratio, there would appear to be little if any relation between altitude and fertility when ethnic composition is controlled. Other factors affecting fecundity, such as nutrition, venereal disease, and so on, certainly bear further investigation, but are beyond the scope of this paper.

It is at least plausible that the explanation for fertility differences between the two cultural groups lies in age at contracting unions or in the relative stability of such unions. The only evidence on this matter which can be drawn from the census refers to the incidence of consensual unions. Proportions of mated women aged 15 and over living in consensual unions were computed for all departments and provinces. In the factor analysis, the proportions of mated women in consensual unions show a loading of 0.55 with factor 1, the general fertility factor, and only —0.16 with factor 2, the socioeconomic factor.[7] However, consensual unions show a surprisingly high *positive* correlation with Spanish-speaking (0.47). Consequently, we held the proportions of consensual unions constant and related Spanish-speaking to the child-woman ratio in the 117 provinces. The relation between fertility and consensual unions disappears, but the Spanish-speaking relation is maintained.

National data show a steady decline in consensual unions with age, from 54 percent of current cohabiting unions in age groups 15–19, to 21 percent for women aged 45 and over.[8] It is possible that as time passes mestizo women, feeling more social pressure than Indian women, are more likely to legalize the consensual relations, thus producing greater stability and higher fertility.

[7] Consensual unions seem to be the main component of factor 4, with a loading of 0.50. No other variable has a loading higher than 0.30.

[8] United Nations *Demographic Yearbook*, 1954.

Indeed, the whole complex of findings presented here would be understandable if it could be demonstrated that mestizo groups entered relatively permanent unions earlier than Indian groups and if such unions continued to evidence higher stability over time. While we have no quantitative data on the question at the moment, ethnographic data can provide valuable leads. A survey of monographs on Peruvian communities indicates that there may be very different norms and behavior patterns characteristic of Indian and mestizo cultures.[9]

(1) *In Indian communities premarital relations are expected and pregnancy as a result of such unions results in little social disapproval:*

(a) Among the Aymara " . . . no importance whatever is attached to virginity" (Tschopik).

(b) "Pre-marital sexual freedom is customary in most Quechua communities" (Mishkin).

(c) "Pre-marital sexual relations between young people are accepted and expected. No social stigma is attached to illegitimate children" (Stein).

[9] H. Ghersi Barrera, "El Indígena y el Mestizo en la Comunidad de Marcará," *Revista del Museo Nacional,* Tomo XXIV; J. Gillin, *Moche: A Peruvian Coastal Community* (Smithsonian Institution, 1945); W. Mangin, "The Cultural Significance of the Fiesta Complex in an Indian Hacienda in Peru" (Ph.D. diss., Yale University, 1954); B. Mishkin, "The Contemporary Quechua," in *Handbook of South American Indians,* ed. J. H. Steward, Vol. II (New York: Cooper, 1947); O. Núñez del Prado, *El Hombre y la Familia, su Matrimonio y Organización Político-Social en Q'ero* (Cuzco, 1957); R. Price, "Courtship and Marriage Institutions in Vicos, Peru," Columbia-Cornell-Harvard Field Studies Report, 1961 (mimeo); G. W. Roberts, *The Population of Jamaica* (Cambridge: Cambridge University Press, 1957); J. Snyder, "Group Relations and Social Change in an Andean Village" (Ph.D. diss., Cornell University, 1960); W. Stein, "Hualcán: An Andean Indian Estancia" (Ph.D. diss., Cornell University, 1955); H. Tschopik, *The Aymara of Chucuito Peru* (New York: American Museum of Natural History, 1951); M. Vásquez Varela, "La Antropología Cultural y Nuestro Problema del Indio," *Perú Indígena,* II (June 1952).

(d) ". . . Pre-marital sexual relations are a common occurrence . . . illegitimate children are not a block to marriage for a woman" (Mangin).

(e) "From adolescence to marriage both sexes enjoy complete sexual freedom" (Núñez del Prado).

(2) *In Indian communities marital relationships are relatively unstable:*

(a) "Close to half the women of the village had had children by men other than their husbands." [Of these about a third are now single.] "A number of women never marry but have a series of relationships which never become permanent" (Snyder).

(b) "Aymara matrimony might best be described as 'brittle monogamy.' Marriages are unstable, divorce is easy and frequent" (Tschopik).

(c) ". . . Separation is common" (Mangin).

(d) ". . . Children born from trial marriages are no impediment to the next union of the female" (Vásquez).

(3) In the light of the liberal attitudes toward sex and illegitimacy, *it is not unlikely that cohabiting relationships in Indian communities are contracted fairly late.* Tschopik states that "the Aymara marry late for American Indians. The average age at marriage in Chucuito is 20 for both sexes." A recent investigation of 123 couples in the Indian community of Vicos indicates that the average age at marriage was 23.6 for women, 24.6 for men. Since the average duration of their trial marriage (*watanaki*) was reported to be fifteen months, we deduce that cohabiting relations begin between the ages of 22 and 23 for the female. (Price.)

What reason do we have to believe that the above principles do not apply equally to mestizo communities? Comparable data for mestizo areas are unfortunately less frequent, but indicate a very different attitude toward premarital relations and births out of wedlock. Snyder writes of her community that Indians are "quite aware that an illegitimate child is a major source of scandal among many mestizos, and in talking of townspeople, apply this standard to them." Snyder also makes reference to norms of chaperonage and seclusion of girls in mestizo culture.

In a comparison of Indian and mestizo culture in a Peruvian community, Ghersi notes that the avoidance of premarital relations with one's intended is "especially true among the mestizos" and that "the mestizo woman who has lost her virginity, has pre-marital or extra-marital relations or children out of wedlock is considered 'dishonoured.'"

In the coastal community of Moche, Gillin belittles the norms concerning premarital chastity, but his data show clearly that the norms are in marked contrast to those cited for Indian communities:

"There is a pose taken by most adults that pre-marital intercourse by girls is reprehensible."

"The boy and girl receive a beating if apprehended in the act."

"The modern Peruvian lower-class pattern is followed in requiring that a girl be accompanied by another girl, by a group of boys and girls, or by her parents or brother when she is in public . . . the chaperonage system somewhat restricts promiscuity."

Our hypothesis, then, is that *the permissiveness about sexual relations encourages Indian couples to delay the establishment of cohabiting marital arrangements longer than is characteristic for mestizos, and that cohabiting relationships, once entered into, are less stable than those entered by mestizos.* Such a pattern might have the following consequences for fertility:

(1) Since sexual relations between noncohabiting couples are probably fewer than among cohabiting couples, we might expect young Indian women to be less likely to be mothers than

young mestizo women; but as they become older and enter co-habiting relations this "advantage" would largely disappear.[10] (2) If the cohabiting unions of Indian women are less stable, we would expect higher marital fertility of mestizo women, and the differential would increase over time.

CONCLUSIONS

As early as 1940 substantial differences in fertility between Lima and the rest of the country were apparent when measured by number of births per woman. However, this difference was almost entirely explicable in terms of the lower proportion of Lima women who ever become mothers. The fertility of *mothers* in Lima is only slightly below that of non-Lima mothers. When the 22 departments of Peru are considered, whereas a negative relation between the social variables (urbanization, literacy and Spanish-speaking) and motherhood is apparent, a *positive* relation to the fertility of mothers occurs, especially as regards Spanish-speaking. However, at younger ages women in Spanish-speaking departments are more likely to be mothers, and when urbanization is controlled the relation between motherhood and Spanish-speaking becomes positive. The net result is to produce the highest fertility in Spanish rural areas, the lowest in Indian urban areas.

Based on ethnographic data, these surprising findings were interpreted as due to differential mating patterns on the part of Indian and mestizos. It is suggested that due to more permissive norms concerning sexual relations, Indians establish cohabiting

[10] It is of interest that in the factor analysis the only high loadings with factor 3 are percentage of women aged 15 and over who are mothers, and children per 100 women aged 15 and over. Loadings of these variables for women aged 45 and over are negligible, and the only other relation of any size is the *negative* loading of percentage of women aged 15 and over who are mated. Consequently, we might term the factor "promiscuous early motherhood."

relations later than do mestizos and that such unions are less stable than mestizo unions, even though common law relations are more characteristic in Spanish-speaking areas.

At least one other possible explanation is that underreporting of births is more characteristic of Indian-speaking areas. However, we would expect the same to be true for rural areas, but in fact, higher motherhood rates (but not mother fertility) were reported for rural areas.

Further validation of the hypotheses developed here must await analyses of the 1961 census and a sample survey conducted by the writer.[11] If the foregoing interpretations are correct, however, an important implication emerges.

Closure of the "demographic gap" in certain countries in Latin America may be longer in coming than had been expected. Increasing modernization may, at least in the short run, increase the fertility of Indian groups by bringing their mating patterns more in line with those of mestizo cultures. Further, if lower rates of fertility in urban areas are in fact due to a lower incidence of mating rather than to the conscious control of fertility within marriage, improved economic circumstances in urban areas may increase fertility by lowering the age at marriage.[12] The practical importance of such possibilities, as well as the general significance for demographic theory, argues for much closer attention to social and cultural aspects of mating and fertility than has been characteristic of Latin American demography.

[11] See J. M. Stycos, "Differential Fertility in Lima, Peru," *Proceedings of the 1961 International Population Union Conference* (London: John Wright and Sons, 1963).

[12] For elaboration on the hypothesis for the Caribbean, see J. Blake et al., *Family Structure in Jamaica* (New York: Free Press, 1961); G. W. Roberts, *The Population of Jamaica* (Cambridge: Cambridge University Press, 1957); J. M. Stycos, *Familia y Fecundidad en Puerto Rico* (México: Fondo de Cultura Económica, 1958); and J. M. Stycos and K. W. Back, *The Control of Human Fertility in Jamaica* (Ithaca, N.Y.: Cornell University Press, 1964).

APPENDIX
(Tables 58–61)

Table 58. Births per 100 women by age, residence and Spanish-speaking (unweighted means, 22 departments)

Age	Rural-Indian	Rural-Spanish	Urban-Spanish
15–19	12	19	18
20–24	96	126	119
25–29	220	270	253
30–34	346	402	386
35–39	443	519	512
40–44	512	589	574
45–49	551	619	611
50 and over	548	560	593
Number	(8)	(6)	(8)

Table 59. Various fertility measures by child-woman ratio (unweighted means, 22 departments)

Child-woman ratios	Mean births per 100 women aged 15 and over	Mean births per 100 women aged 45 and over	Mean births per 100 mothers aged 15 and over	Number of departments
–78	260	490	476	(2)
78–85	319	532	484	(9)
86–92	340	547	487	(3)
93–104	380	625	535	(5)
105+	369	667	532	(3)

233

Table 60. Pearsonian correlation coefficients, 12 demographic and social variables for 22 departments of Peru, 1940

Variables	2	3	4	5	6	7	8	9	10	11	12
1 Child-woman ratio	0.45	0.44	0.59	0.70	0.55	0.61	0.51	0.43	-0.05	-0.39	0.22
2 Percentage women aged 15 and over who are mothers		0.70	0.85	0.39	0.25	0.12	0.14	0.27	-0.53	-0.61	-0.26
3 Percentage women aged 45 and over who are mothers			0.70	0.53	0.26	0.13	0.14	0.05	-0.44	-0.49	-0.27
4 Births per 100 women aged 15 and over				0.76	0.69	0.59	0.36	0.45	-0.20	-0.33	0.08
5 Births per 100 women aged 45 and over					0.91	0.90	0.52	0.52	0.21	0.02	0.40
6 Births per 100 mothers aged 15 and over						0.94	0.50	0.46	0.29	0.17	0.48
7 Births per 100 mothers aged 45 and over							0.54	0.58	0.47	0.26	0.61
8 Percentage women aged 15 and over currently mated								0.38	-0.02	-0.14	0.08
9 Percentage of mated in common law unions									0.20	-0.05	0.47
10 Percentage literate										0.88	0.80
11 Percentage urban											0.57
12 Percentage Spanish-speaking only											—

234

Table 61. Factor analysis of twelve variables, 22 departments of Peru, 1940 (rotated matrix)[a]

Variables	Factor I	Factor II	Factor III	Factor IV
1 Child-woman ratio	0.73	−0.30	−0.08	−0.21
2 Percentage women aged 15 and over who are mothers	0.38	−0.64	−0.61	0.07
3 Percentage women aged 45 and over who are mothers	0.42	−0.58	0.30	−0.31
4 Births per 100 women aged 15 and over	0.75	−0.35	0.52	0.01
5 Births per 100 women aged 45 and over	0.96	0.01	0.04	−0.14
6 Births per 100 mothers aged 15 and over	0.94	0.16	0.02	−0.08
7 Births per 100 mothers aged 45 and over	0.94	0.31	−0.10	0.09
8 Percentage women aged 15 and over currently mated	0.56	−0.16	−0.34	0.19
9 Percentage of mated in common law unions	0.55	0.10	0.11	0.50
10 Percentage literate	0.21	0.92	−0.01	0.06
11 Percentage urban	−0.01	0.94	0.02	−0.19
12 Percentage Spanish-speaking only	0.43	0.72	0.06	0.28

[a] Factored by the Complete Centroid Method; rotated by the Quarti-max Method. See F. Neuhaus and C. Wrigley, "The Quartimax Method," *British Journal of Statistical Psychology*, VII (November 1954).

15

Female Employment and
Fertility in Lima, Peru

With rising levels of education, urbanization, and industrialization, modernizing areas can anticipate that increasing numbers of women will enter the labor force. A popular hypothesis among demographers suggests that the employment of females in nonagricultural occupations depresses fertility. Moreover, such a belief is frequently voiced by policy makers in modernizing areas, and helps to rationalize their failure to initiate direct measures of fertility control.

A recent ecological analysis based on Peruvian census data of 1940 revealed that among the twenty-one nonmetropolitan departments, completed fertility showed a fairly high negative correlation with female employment. The author concludes that "female labor force participation in Peru reduces fertility by reducing the fertility of married women. . . . The use of some birth control method allows married women to work. On the other hand, the necessity to work encourages the conscious control of births."[1]

The data used in the above-mentioned study are subject to the usual limitations of ecological data. Moreover, even if a relation between fertility and employment exists, we may question the assumption that birth control practices are motivated by the

[1] David M. Heer, "Fertility Differences between Indian and Spanish-Speaking Parts of Andean Countries," *Population Studies*, 18, 79–80, (July 1964).

desire to work. Certainly if such a direct relation exists, we would expect that it would be most apparent in urban areas. Various kinds of data from recent urban studies in Peru raise doubts concerning a direct and general causal relation between female employment and fertility.

For the city of Lima all 1959 birth registration data were punched on IBM cards by the Servicio Cooperativo Interamericano de Salud Publica (SCISP), and special tabulations were prepared for the writer. Since population base data were not available, our measure of fertility is live birth order, by age of mother.

While the fertility of office workers is markedly lower than that of other mothers, the fertility of service workers is virtually identical with that of the nonemployed. (See Table 62.) However, the former group constitutes less than 4 percent of the employed mothers, the latter over two-thirds. Thus while certain female occupations show very low relative fertility, being

Table 62. Index numbers for mean birth order, by age and occupation of mother (nonemployed mothers = 100)

Age	Office workers	Professional and technical	Artisans and factory workers	Service workers	Nonemployed
15–19	86	93	92	104	100
20–24	64	91	83	100	100
25–29	54	85	88	99	100
30–34	52	84	88	97	100
35–39	51	82	98	99	100
Age standardized mean birth order	2.00	3.01	3.13	3.47	3.51
Percent in occupational category	2	13	4	43	36

in the labor force per se, especially where this means service occupations, does not necessarily imply lower fertility in Lima. Indeed, since most urban employment opportunities for women are in service occupations, there are no grounds for optimism concerning the effects of urban employment on fertility.

The foregoing data deal only with fertile women. There is, of course, the possibility that many working women never marry or never have children.[2] The sample survey of currently mated Lima women aged 20–44 conducted by the writer in 1960 and 1961 can provide further evidence on at least the marital fertility of employed and unemployed women, although type of employment was not recorded in the inquiry.

Since no census had been taken in Peru since 1940, it was not possible, with the resources available, to draw a refined probability sample. Consequently, a procedure was adopted which probably resulted in certain biases: (1) The city's 4,454 blocks were numbered and ninety blocks were chosen at random. Interviewers then proceeded in a systematic fashion to visit from house to house in the selected blocks until twenty eligible women were interviewed, yielding a total of about 1,800 interviews. This procedure probably caused an overrepresentation of upper-class subjects, who are more likely to live on blocks with small populations. (2) Since the slum areas (*barriadas*) were inadequately mapped, a special sample representing 10 percent of the total sample was taken. This proportion was decided on by the Carlos A. Uriarte Market Research Associates in Lima, based on various estimates of the population of Lima and the *barriadas*. From 128 *barriadas* judged to be in the metropolitan area, 10 were chosen at random, rough maps were drawn, and 20 cases were located by house-to-house canvassing. Some local observers believe 10 percent to be an underestimate of the *barriada* proportion.

[2] According to the 1940 census of Peru, Lima women do have much higher rates of childlessness than women in the remainder of the country. See Chapter 14.

Another source of bias may stem from the large number of eligible women not interviewed. Over 5,000 canvass or prelist visits were required in order to secure the 1,995 interviews contained in the final sample. In 8 percent of the visits the house was found to be unoccupied or to be a business establishment; in just under one-third, there was no one eligible for interview; another 4 percent refused to be canvassed, and we have no information on 6.5 percent of the canvass visits. In the remaining 50 percent of the canvass visits, an eligible woman was found to be living in the household. However, in 21 percent of these 2,541 households known to contain a woman eligible for interview, interviews were not actually carried out, largely because of refusals (39 percent) and failure to find respondent at home after two call-backs (38 percent). Another 10 percent of eligibles not interviewed were temporarily elsewhere (e.g., on vacation); assorted reasons and no information comprise the remaining 12 percent. (See Table 63.)

These are much higher rates than experienced in earlier studies by the author in the Caribbean[3] and call for some explanation. First, previous studies were restricted to lower-class women and it is clear from the data in Table 63 that upper-class districts in Lima showed far higher rates of refusal and failure to be contacted than did other areas of the city. Even the brief canvass interview to determine eligibility for interviews showed a refusal rate in the upper-class districts over three times as high as those in other districts.

Upper-class women were not only less likely to be at home than lower-class women, but even when at home they often used the servant to keep the interviewer away. One of the major and more satisfying roles of the servant in the upper-class home is that of gatekeeper. The following are typical comments written by interviewers:

[3] J. Mayone Stycos, "The Sample Survey for Social Science in Underdeveloped Areas," in Richard Adams and Jack Preiss, eds., *Human Organization Research* (Homewood, Ill.: The Dorsey Press, Inc., 1960).

Table 63. Rates of refusal and noncontact, Lima (in percent)

Subjects	Upper-class[a] districts	Other districts
Women known to be eligible for interviews who were not interviewed	34	17
Noninterviewed eligibles who refused interview	37	41
All eligibles who refused interview	13	7
All canvass contacts made who refused to be canvassed	7	2
All contacts made (canvass and interview) who refused interview or canvass	13	5

[a] San Isidro and Miraflores.

The servant always came out saying that the lady of the house was not in and that she [the servant] did not know how to answer the questions.

The lady of the house did not appear, but sent her servant to close the door.

I couldn't speak with the lady of the house personally. The servant transmitted the message and the answer was negative.

Even when the lady of the house herself appeared, her social class and sophistication made it much easier for her than for lower-class respondents to refuse to answer questions. Occasionally the sophistication reached unusual levels!

The lady explained that she had read Dr. Stycos' book on Puerto Rico and discussed it with her husband. She had no desire to participate in such studies.

The interviewers were young, inexperienced, and rarely from upper-class families. They were often more terrified of the upper-class districts than of the fearsome slums of Lima.

Thus we emerge with the suspicion that the upper classes are not only overrepresented in the sample, but that those who are represented may not be entirely typical of their class because of the high nonresponse rate. In an attempt to assess the nature of the latter bias, supervisors were sent back to do a subsample of 150 cases who, for one reason or another, had not been interviewed; but these data have not yet been analyzed. To adjust for the possible class bias, we have held social class constant throughout the paper.[4]

Twenty percent of the sampled Lima women had worked throughout the previous year and an additional 7 percent had worked for part of it.[5] In this paper these groups are merged and classified as "working." Working status shows some relation to social class, with 18 percent of the top class, 29 percent of the middle-class, and 36 percent of the lower-class women reporting that they had worked at some time during the past year.[6]

It is, first of all, of interest to note in Table 64 that age at first union is higher for working women only among those of the highest class. Second, there is a negative relation between employment and absolute number of children for the highest and lowest social classes, and a weak but similar relation among the middle groups. If we examine percentages working by number of live births, however, we find that the relationship is by no means a continuous one. Figure 1 shows that in each class a sharp drop in percentages working occurs after the birth of one or two children, but that from this point on the number of children bears no relation to employment status. Thus women with eight or more children are just as likely (or more likely) to be working as those with three or four.

Our study of Jamaican fertility found a close relation between

[4] Interviewers were requested to categorize the respondent's social class level in one of four groups. See Table 16, p. 148.

[5] The question asked was: "Did you work for pay at all during the past year?"

[6] Education shows a similar negative relation to employment, up to the university level. Those with some university training (about 5 percent of the sample) have as high an incidence of employment as those with less than three years education (38 percent).

241

Table 64. Various demographic characteristics by socioeconomic[a] and employment status

	Class A		Class B		Class C	
	Working	Not working	Working	Not working	Working	Not working
Mean live births	2.4	3.0	3.6	3.8	4.0	4.6
Mean living children	2.3	2.9	3.3	3.5	3.5	4.1
Live births per 1,000 mated years[b]	264	271	305	340	336	420
Living children per 1,000 mated years	252	267	281	317	289	374
Mean age	32.1	32.7	32.2	31.4	31.0	30.0
Mean years education	7.5	7.0	4.0	4.4	2.5	2.5
Mean age 1st union	22.9	21.9	20.0	20.1	19.2	19.3
Mean mated years	9.0	11.0	11.9	11.2	12.0	10.9
Number of cases	(132)	(611)	(222)	(535)	(190)	(315)

[a] Socioeconomic status was determined by the interviewers who rated the household as A, B, C, or D. As seen in Table 16, sharp distinctions of education, age, expenditures, and fertility occur among the three lowest classes but not between the two highest classes. Classes A and B have been merged and termed "A" for purposes of the present analysis.

[b] Mated years are derived by subtracting age at first cohabiting union from current age.

fertility, marital status, and employment, the evidence supporting the hypothesis that legal marriage (as opposed to common law arrangements) depresses the level of female employment

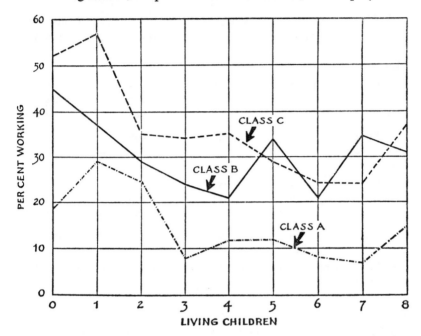

Figure 1. Percent of females who worked in past year, by number of living children for each of three socioeconomic classes, Lima

and also raises fertility.[7] Table 65 shows that consensually married women are much more likely to be employed than legally married women within each fertility and socioeconomic category. It is still the case that women of higher fertility are less likely to be working, but we see again that the sharpest break occurs after the birth of one child.

We believe, however, that women with 0–2 births in Peru, especially in the lower economic classes, are unlikely to be practicing birth control. Should this be the case it might suggest that low fertility encourages or permits a woman to work. Since

[7] J. Mayone Stycos and Kurt W. Back, *The Control of Human Fertility in Jamaica* (Ithaca, N.Y.: Cornell University Press, 1964).

Table 65. Employment status, by number of living children, socioeconomic and marital status[a]

Class	Percent working		Number	
	Married	Consensual union	Married	Consensual union
Middle				
0–1	35	50	104	40
2–3	24	39	237	54
4+	25	35	257	65
Total	26	40	598	159
Lower				
0–1	51	59	39	44
2–3	27	51	109	53
4+	27	43	185	65
Total	30	50	333	162

[a] The incidence of common law unions among the upper class was too low for inclusion in this table.

we did not ask about contraceptive practices in the sample, we must look to less direct data. If employment were antecedent to fertility we would expect that the relation would be strongest in the upper classes, where birth control is more likely to be practiced, and that working and nonworking women would show very different attitudes with respect to desired number of children.

We have already seen that, in terms of absolute number of children, the upper-class working women have 20 percent fewer living children than nonworking women, the lower-class working women have 15 percent fewer, and middle-class women have 5 percent fewer. However, the different categories have somewhat different average lengths of marriage. When we relate the number of live births to years mated, we find that the fertility of working and nonworking women in the upper class is virtually identical; that the middle-class working women have

only 10 percent lower fertility rates; and that lower-class working women have 20 percent lower rates than nonworking
women. Thus, the class in which we would expect a "career
orientation" to lead to direct measures for voluntary control
shows no evidence of differential fertility by employment status,
whereas the lowest class shows a substantial differential.

Now let us see whether employment is related to attitudes
toward family size, on the assumption that if working status
motivates lower fertility in a direct way it must operate through
the medium of attitudes.

Table 66 shows no consistent relation between working status
and ideal number of children when class and number of children
are controlled. On the other hand, a more consistent positive
relation emerges between ideal size of family and living children,
and between ideal size and social class.

Table 66. Median ideal number of living children, by employment
status, social class, and number of living children

Class	Working	Not working
Upper		
0–1	3.3	3.2
2–3	3.4	3.2
4 +	4.0	4.2
Middle		
0–1	3.2	2.8
2–3	3.2	3.3
4 +	3.4	3.7
Lower		
0–1	2.3	2.6
2–3	3.0	3.5
4 +	3.7	3.2

Table 67 presents responses to the question: "Do you want
any more children than you now have?" Among women with
four or more children, the working women in each class are
more likely to desire no additional children. However, with two

to three children there is no relation, and for women of very low fertility, precisely those most likely to be working, there is the suggestion of a positive relation between employment and desire for more children among the two extreme classes.

Table 67. Percent desiring no more children, by social class, number of living children, and employment status

Class	Working	Not working
Upper		
0–1	4	10
2–3	36	33
4+	68	51
Middle		
0–1	18	16
2–3	31	35
4+	69	62
Lower		
0–1	15	24
2–3	45	41
4+	71	60

We might further expect working women to be more sensitive to the economic implications of an additional child, but from Table 68 we see that only among the upper class are working women more sensitive, the class in which fertility rates were virtually identical.

Finally, in terms of degree of concern about family size, we asked whether the women had ever thought about how many children they wanted to have, and, if they had thought about it, whether they had ever discussed it with their husbands. From Table 69 we see that social class and fertility, but not employment, relate to the degree of preoccupation about size of the family.

Lima is considered to be an old conservative city, with traditional occupations and traditional ideas. We therefore repeated

Table 68. Mean economic sensitivity score by social class, employment status, and number of living children[a]

Class	Working	Not working
Upper		
0–1	1.9	2.3
2–3	1.5	1.7
4 +	1.1	1.7
Middle		
0–1	1.6	1.6
2–3	1.3	1.3
4 +	1.2	1.1
Lower		
0–1	1.5	1.3
2–3	1.2	1.2
4 +	1.0	1.0

[a] The score ranges from 0 to 3; the higher the score the less the sensitivity to the economic impact of an additional child.

0 = One more child would affect respondent's economic condition a lot.

1 = Three more children would affect respondent's economic condition a lot.

2 = Three more children would affect respondent's economic condition a little.

3 = Three more children would not affect respondent's economic condition.

the survey in Chimbote, a city which has experienced extremely high rates of population growth because of opportunities for employment in the steel and fish-canning industries. Most employed women are working in small factories. The "untraditional" character of the city and its unique female labor force should provide an interesting contrast to Lima.

The patterns described in Lima are even more clear-cut in Chimbote. Although working women have a smaller average number of children, on all the attitude questions there are no differences between working and nonemployed women, except in the case of preferred family size. In this instance working

Table 69. Mean score of preoccupation about family size,[a] by socio-economic status, number of living children, and employment status

Class	Working	Not working
Upper		
0–1	1.4	1.5
2–3	1.3	1.3
4 +	1.0	1.0
Middle		
0–1	1.0	1.0
2–3	0.8	0.8
4 +	0.5	0.8
Lower		
0–1	0.7	0.7
2–3	0.7	0.6
4 +	0.6	0.4

[a] 0 = Have not thought; 1 = Thought but not talked to husband; 2 = Talked to husband.

women consistently express preferences for somewhat larger families. It is the case, however, that working women in each economic class started their first marital union later than non-working women.

SUMMARY

Using 1959 Lima birth registration data it was found that mean birth order by age of mother is virtually identical for housewives and service workers, the latter constituting two-thirds of the female labor force. Mothers classified in professional and technical categories showed about 14 percent fewer births and office workers 43 percent fewer. Office workers, however, represent less than 4 percent of the female labor force. A recent survey of currently mated women in Lima shows no clear-cut relation between fertility and employment status. In each social class, women with 0–2 children are more likely to be working than women with more children, but the proportions working do not diminish after about three children. Further, in terms of fertility rates, the strongest relation is characteristic of the lowest economic class, where birth control is least likely to be practiced. In the upper class, no differences in fertility rate by employment status were found.

This suggested that whatever relation exists between number of children and employment is not due to conscious controls on fertility. To test this hypothesis attitudes of working and nonworking women toward family size were compared.

Few consistent differences emerged, other than the fact that in the upper class working women have somewhat higher sensitivity than nonworking women to the economic effects of additional children, and that working women with four or more living children are less likely than others to want additional children. They are, however, no more likely to have thought about the matter before or to have discussed it with their husbands. When the foregoing analysis was repeated for the rapidly growing industrial city of Chimbote, attitudes were even more homogeneous; however, age at first union was somewhat higher for working women in each class. It seems likely, therefore, that employment status is more often a consequence of marital fertility than a cause. It is also likely that legal marriage reduces female employment and at the same time increases fertility by stabilizing sexual relationships. The present analysis gives little comfort to Peruvians who are hoping for increased entry of females into the labor force as a solution to high birth rates.

16

Education and Fertility
in Latin America

Latin American countries invest fairly heavily in education, in one way or another. Toward the end of the fifties, six countries were expending $10.00 or more per capita per year on education: in order of descending magnitude—Venezuela, Brazil, Panama, Colombia, Costa Rica, and Chile.[1] No country was expending less than 8 percent of its total public spending on education, and four were spending more than a fifth. Such outlays for education represented from 1.2 percent of the national income in Colombia to as much as 4 percent in Peru.

The most common justification for such expenditures relates to the role of education in economic and social modernization, but in addition it is sometimes alleged that education will have a pay-off in reduced fertility levels. With increasing education, birth rates are expected "automatically" to decline, obviating the necessity for direct programs of fertility control. To test this assumption we have assembled three classes of data on the relation of fertility to education in Latin America—international, interregional (intranational), and interpersonal.

NATIONAL DATA

There are two general types of educational measures available for Latin America: those which reflect current success at edu-

[1] *Statistical Abstract of Latin America, 1962,* Table 14, p. 25.

cating the present generation of children (e.g., proportion of school-age population currently enrolled in primary or secondary schools), and those which reflect earlier success at education (measures of the total or adult population such as the proportion who have had a primary school education). The pattern of intercorrelation of these measures substantiates the distinctions (Table 70). While the variables of mean years of schooling and the ratio of postprimary to primary school among the adult

Table 70. Intercorrelation of educational measures for 18–20 Latin American countries, around 1950

Educational measures	A	B	C	D
A. Mean years of schooling[a]	—	—	—	—
B. Population with postprimary education per 100 with primary[a]	.92	—	—	—
C. Percent 5–14 in primary school	.23	.10	—	—
D. Percent 5–14 in secondary school	.45	.16	.68	—
E. Percent illiterate[a]	−.40	−.08	−.85	−.70

[a] Population aged 15 and over.

Source: Original measures reported by Oscar Vera, "The Educational Situation and Requirement in Latin America," in E. DeVries and J. Echevarría, eds., *Social Aspects of Economic Development in Latin America* (UNESCO, 1963).

population are closely related, they show little relation to measures of the school-age population. Literacy appears more closely related to measures of the school-age population than to measures of the adult population.

Thus Argentina, Costa Rica, and Cuba, whose illiteracy rates average only 19 percent, have only about ten persons with postprimary school education for every hundred with primary schooling. On the other hand, Chile, Panama, and Puerto Rico, while also countries of low illiteracy (averaging 26 percent), have much higher postprimary school ratios—an average of 38 percent. The absence of correlation between these two measures is a particularly interesting one, suggesting that some countries may have concentrated on mass education at a low level at the expense of postprimary schooling, others at training a fairly large educational elite while neglecting the mass of the population. In some cases it may be that education for the masses is just beginning and the next decade will see the large wave of primary-school educated pass through the secondary system. The implications for national fertility rates could be very different depending on which way education is distributed in the population. Since the measures of education for adult and school-age populations are poorly correlated, we would expect fertility to be related to the former rather than the latter, if education effects fertility declines.

To test this thesis, we correlated various measures of fertility with the educational measures cited above. For twenty Latin American countries (including Puerto Rico and excluding Uruguay), the child-woman ratio was available as a measure of fertility, and for eight countries the crude birth rate, general fertility rate and total fertility rate were available. For the remaining countries, estimates based on Bogue and Palmore's techniques are used.[2]

Fairly high correlations are found, especially with the crude birth rate, where 40 to 50 percent of the variance can be accounted for by variations in literacy or percent in secondary schools (Table 71). The correlations are higher for the eight countries judged to have good census and vital statistics data, and lower for other countries.

[2] See Jay Cho, "Estimated Refined Measures of Fertility for all Major Countries of the World," *Demography*, I, No. 1 (1964); and D. J. Bogue and J. A. Palmore, "Some Empirical and Analytic Relations Among Demographic Fertility Measures, with Regression Models for Fertility Estimation," *ibid.*

Table 71. Correlation between educational variables and fertility in 20 Latin American countries, around 1950

Fertility measures	Percent illiterate	Percent 5–14 in primary	Percent 5–14 in secondary	Mean years schooling	Post-primary ratio
Child-woman ratio	.33	−.31	−.41	−.29	−.18
Crude birth rate	.61	−.62	−.70	−.51	−.31
General fertility rate	.51	−.52	−.63	−.46	−.30
Total fertility rate	.48	−.48	−.60	−.40	−.27

Sources: Educational measures from O. Vera, *op. cit.* Fertility rates from Lee Jay Cho, "Estimated Refined Measures of Fertility for all Major Countries of the World," *op. cit.*

But contrary to our expectation, there is a tendency, especially marked for countries with deficient data, for fertility to be related more strongly to the educational measures of the *school-age* population or to literacy (which was seen to be closely related) than to the measures more heavily influenced by the adult population, the mean years of schooling, and the post-primary school ratio.

The high correlations with current rather than past educational efforts suggest that the relationship may be the consequence of other variables related both to fertility and recent educational attainments. One of the more obvious relevant variables is urbanization, which, as measured by the proportion of population living in places of 20,000 population or more, has a correlation of −.77 with illiteracy, and −.80 with the crude birth rate. The partial correlation of illiteracy and the birth rate drops to .03 when urbanization is controlled, but that between urbanization and the birth rate declines only to −.65 when illiteracy is controlled. (If child-woman ratios rather than birth rates are used, the respective partials are −.37 and −.67.) International fertility variations, then, are largely accounted for by urbanization rather than by education.

REGIONAL DATA

Now let us look at intranational variations. For eleven of the Latin American countries we have computed child-woman ratios, percent literate, and proportions urban for each of the political subunits of the nation around 1950. In the case of all countries but Bolivia the relation of literacy and fertility is negative, though under —.20 in Panama, Mexico, and Honduras (Table 72). Again, however, in all countries, the relation of urbanization and literacy is positive. When urbanization is held constant by partial correlation, the literacy-fertility relation remains high primarily in those countries with the highest educational development—Argentina, Chile, and Costa Rica. In most of the remaining countries the sign is reversed or the relation approaches zero. In the case of each of ten countries, we divided the subunits into those with high and those with low proportions urban (the cutting point at the median) and recomputed the literacy-fertility correlations within each of the groups.

We see again from Table 72 that only in the countries with the highest educational levels—Argentina, Chile, and Costa Rica —does the negative relation between literacy and fertility hold in both "rural" and "urban" provinces. Among the less urban provinces as many countries show positive relations between literacy and fertility as negative. Even among the more urbanized provinces the relation is positive in three countries, though in two of them it is quite weak. Thus, among the countries we have considered, a general literacy-fertility relation is confined to countries of high educational attainments, but in most of the remaining countries is restricted to the more urbanized regions of the nation.

Table 72. Intercorrelations of literacy, child-woman ratios and urbanization for the political subunits of 11 Latin American countries, around 1950

Countries	Fertility ratio	Percent urban	Correlations of percent literate with:			Number of units
			Child-woman ratio holding percent urban constant	Child-woman ratio in areas with high percent urban	Child-woman ratio in areas with low percent urban	
Argentina	-.74	.27	-.74	-.71	-.77	24
Bolivia	.50	.32	.40	.84	.83	9
Chile	-.78	.85	-.46	-.81	-.55	25
Colombia	-.36	.34	-.31	—	—	24
Costa Rica	-.60	.33	-.55	-.59	-.52	65
Guatemala	-.46	.68	.03	-.77	.29	22
Honduras	-.16	.66	-.06	.29	-.73	16
Mexico	-.20	.63	.28	-.47	.39	32
Nicaragua	-.60	.89	.16	-.29	.58	17
Panama	-.10	.45	.27	.27	-.46	64
Venezuela	-.25	.88	.21	-.41	.49	23

Source: National censuses; computations by International Population Program.

DATA ON INDIVIDUALS

Direct data—that is, the cross-tabulation of fertility and educational characteristics of individuals—are scarce for Latin America. Preliminary data from the urban fertility surveys in Bogotá, Caracas, Mexico City, Panama City, Rio de Janeiro and San José show that women with no education have had from two and a half to almost four times as many live births as women with some university education. The pattern of the decline is by no means regular from city to city. In two there is virtually no difference in fertility between those with no education and those with four or five years; whereas in two others it exceeds 25 percent. Again, in three cities the difference in births between those who have completed secondary school and those who have attended the university is less than 25 percent, but in two others it exceeds 60 percent. However, no controls, such as age, have been introduced. (In Santiago, Chile, a tabulation for women aged 35–50 showed that women required six years of primary school before having one child less than women with one year of schooling or less.[3]) Nevertheless, the overall relation appears strong in each city. Since data for *rural* areas are not available for these countries, we turn to survey data from Peru and census data from Puerto Rico.

Peru

In Peru, Chapters 10 and 15 have introduced the survey carried out in four types of Peruvian communities: the metropolis of

[3] From survey data reported in C. A. Miró and F. Rath, "Preliminary Findings of Comparative Fertility Surveys in Three Latin American Countries," *Milbank Memorial Fund Quarterly*, XLIII (October 1965), and L. Tabah and R. Samuel, "Preliminary Findings of a Survey of Fertility and Attitudes Toward Family Formation in Santiago, Chile," in C. V. Kiser, ed., *Research in Family Planning* (Princeton: Princeton University Press, 1962).

Lima, a provincial city of extraordinary population growth (Chimbote), a highland town (Huaylas), and a coastal village (Virú). Because of the small number of women interviewed in Virú, and because of their similarity in low levels of education and income, the cases from Virú and Huaylas have been grouped for the present analysis.

Mean number of live births by the time of the survey was lowest in Lima (3.6), highest in Virú and Huaylas (4.7), and at the high level of 4.4 in Chimbote. To what extent are the differences in fertility due to the differences in education of the women? Table 73 shows the mean number of live births standardized for age, for various educational levels in the three areas. Several generalizations may be drawn:

Table 73. Mean live births (cumulative fertility ratios) standardized for age,[a] by education and place of residence, currently mated women, Peru

Years of education	Lima	Chimbote	Virú-Huaylas
0	4.7	5.1	5.0
1–2	4.4	5.2	4.3
3–4	4.3	5.3	4.2
5	3.5	4.2[b]	4.1[b]
1–4 secondary	3.3	—[c]	—
Completed secondary	2.5	—	—
Number of cases	(1,993)	(623)	(450)

[a] Direct standardization, Lima age distribution.
[b] Women who completed primary school or more.
[c] Dash indicates insufficient number of cases for age breakdown.

(1) Education has a negative relation to fertility in all three areas, but the relation is most regular and pronounced in the metropolis of Lima.

(2) Holding education constant does not eliminate the fertility differentials between Lima and Huaylas-Virú prior to fifth

year of education. (Here we must consider the possibility of greater underreporting of births by the rural women of four or less years of education, but this aspect has not yet been analyzed.)

(3) In the cities, fertility shows little or no decline prior to five years of education, after which the decline is precipitous. In Virú and Huaylas, however, those with no education have higher fertility than those with one or two years.

Table 74 provides further insight into the nature of differentials. Age at first marriage (or consensual union) is shown to bear a positive relation to education, and in Chimbote does not appear

Table 74. Mean age at first marital union, by education and place of residence, Peru

Years of education	Lima	Chimbote	Virú-Huaylas
0	18.2	20.5	18.6
1	18.7	19.8	19.3
2	19.4	19.8	19.7
3	19.6	19.4	20.5
4	20.0	18.4	20.1
5–6	20.4	20.7	20.6
1–2 secondary	20.7	21.7	22.2[a]
3–4 secondary	21.8	22.2	—[b]
Completed secondary	22.5	23.7	—

[a] Some secondary schooling or beyond (12 cases).
[b] Dash indicates less than 12 cases.

at all until secondary school. Lima women appear to marry slightly *earlier* than women in the other areas. Thus, variation in age at marriage may help to account for the fertility differentials between educational categories but not between residence categories.

In Table 75, the major effects of age-at-marriage differentials are eliminated by confining our data to women aged 35 and over; and by expressing fertility in terms of births per year of marriage.

Table 75. Live births per hundred exposure years,[a] by education and place of residence, women 35 and over, Peru

Years of education	Lima	Chimbote	Virú-Huaylas
0	29.9	41.2	33.7
1–2	31.7	45.8	35.6
3–4	30.6	46.7	37.9
5	25.1	35.8	33.8[b]
1–4 Secondary	23.4	38.5[c]	—[d]
Completed secondary	22.2	—	—
Number of Cases	(699)	(177)	(202)

[a] Since education is positively related to age at marriage, it is negatively related to years of exposure. The range of mean years of exposure for Lima women is from 19.3 for women of no education to 15.4 for those with some high school. A similar range is found in Virú-Huaylas, but hardly any in Chimbote.

[b] Women who completed primary school or more (31 cases).

[c] Women with one year of secondary school or more (16 cases).

[d] Dash indicates insufficient number of cases for analysis.

This procedure increases the differences in fertility among the three areas, while the differentials according to educational level prior to the end of primary school virtually disappear. Indeed, outside of Lima it is difficult to say that there is any relation between education and fertility at all, since the fertility of the best educated women in each area is little different from that of the least educated.

That some form of voluntary restriction of fertility is responsible for the differences may be deduced from Figure 2. Part A of the figure refers to the average number of live births borne in the first five years of marriage to all women who have completed at least five years of marriage. In the first five years of marriage there is no variation in number of live births either among areas or among educational groups—everyone has just under two births. (This would minimize the importance of biological or climatic factors as explanations of differences between areas.)

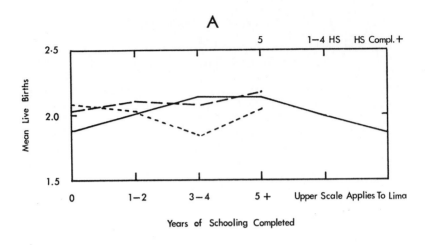

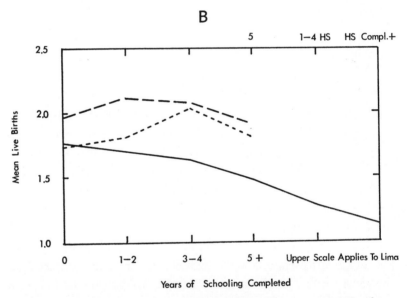

Figure 2. Mean live births in successive completed five-year intervals of marriage, by education, for three places of residence, Peru

A. First five-year interval since marriage
B. Second interval (5th through 9th year of marriage)   — Lima
C. Third interval (10th through 14th year of marriage)   – – Chimbote
D. Fourth interval (15th through 19th year of marriage)   - - - Virú-Huaylas

C

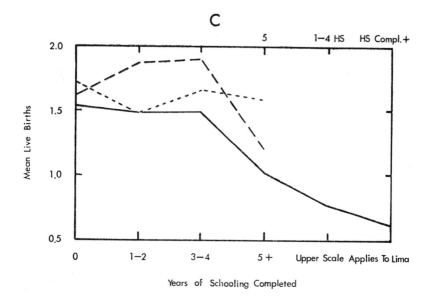

5   1—4 HS   HS Compl.+

Mean Live Births

2.0

1.5

1.0

0.5

0   1—2   3—4   5 +   Upper Scale Applies To Lima

Years of Schooling Completed

D

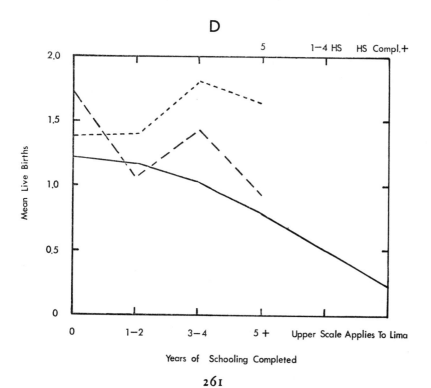

5   1—4 HS   HS Compl.+

Mean Live Births

2.0

1.5

1.0

0.5

0

0   1—2   3—4   5 +   Upper Scale Applies To Lima

Years of Schooling Completed

261

Part B of the Figure 2 refers to the mean number of live births which occurred in the second five years of marriage to all women who have completed at least ten years of marriage. During the second five years, Lima women begin to have fewer births than others, and education beyond the fourth year begins to be related to lower fertility. This tendency is magnified in Lima in the third and fourth five-year intervals, but in the other areas the relation to education is not clear (Figure 2, Parts C and D). In Chimbote, a slight decline for the upper educational groups may be emerging, but only after the third and fourth five-year periods of marriage.

We infer, then, that even women of little or no education are controlling their fertility in Lima—perhaps by abortion, although the net effect is not great. Increasing doses of education have little effect until the end of primary school in Lima, and in the other areas the relation is minimal and can be explained by age at marriage.

Puerto Rico

The case of Puerto Rico is especially interesting since it has shown remarkable gains in education over the past half-century. According to census data, 55 percent of its population over age 10 was illiterate in 1920, 41 percent in 1930, 32 percent in 1940, 25 percent in 1950, and 19 percent in 1960. The birth rate, however, showed no signs of change until the turn of the half-century, when it began dropping from about 40 to its present rate of about 31. However, other evidence indicates that much of this decline was due to the out-migration of Puerto Ricans in the reproductive ages. It would appear that major improvements in education do not produce automatic fertility declines within the time span discussed.

Utilizing 1955 sample survey data from the Puerto Rican Bureau of Labor Statistics, A. Jaffe concludes that "at least six and possibly nine years of schooling is required before any significant decline in the birth rate occurs," and "the combined influence of increasing education and increasing participation of women in modern economic enterprises is likely to be more effective than either factor by itself."[4] Jaffe's important thesis that at least six years of schooling were needed in order to have a real influence on fertility was somewhat limited by the broad educational categories reported in his analysis: 0–4 years, 5–9 years, and 10 or more years of schooling. As Jaffe pointed out, "The data do not show at what point the education of women begins to take effect, i.e., whether six, seven, eight or nine years of schooling are needed." Table 76, which utilizes special tabulations from the 1960 census, increases the number of categories. In order to simplify the analysis we have confined the data to legally married women of completed fertility whose spouses are present.

Table 76. Total live births per 1,000 married women aged 45 and over, Puerto Rico, 1960 (legally married with spouses present), by education

Years of school completed	Births per 1000 women	% Change from preceding category	% Women in category
0	7,421	——	35.2
Primary			
1–4	6,896	− 7.0	32.8
5–6	5,836	−15.4	11.7
7–8	4,288	−26.5	8.5
Secondary			
1–3	3,367	−21.5	4.0
4	2,453	−27.1	3.4
College			
1 or more	1,920	−21.7	4.4
Total	6,224		100.0

Source: Special tabulations of the 1960 Census of Puerto Rico.

[4] A. J. Jaffe, People, Jobs and Economic Development (Glencoe: Free Press, 1959), pp. 196–97.

The total range in fertility is very great. Women with no education have had 3.3 times as many births as those with one or more years of college. If the progression were distributed evenly over the approximately fourteen years of education, it would mean that each additional year of schooling produced 0.4 fewer live births—or well over one birth for every three years of schooling. However, the progression is not even. There is a difference of only 7 percent in number of live births between those with no education and those with one to four years. Between the latter category and those with five or six there is a 15 percent reduction in fertility. Thus women with about six years of schooling, a major educational goal for many modernizing countries, have only 1.6 fewer live births by completion of childbearing than women who have had no education. Each year of education over this range means only 0.28 fewer births, and much less than this at the lower end of the educational continuum.

The data indicate an accelerating effect of education on fertility, starting very slowly in the lower primary school[5] and reaching a high level toward the end of junior high school which is maintained thereafter. Differences are especially marked at the points of completing primary school and high school,[6] but from the seventh grade on there are marked differences in fertility with each increment of education.[7]

[5] The accelerating effect of education on fertility may even occur within the 0–4 year category. Published data for ever married women 35–44 (including consensually married, divorced, separated, or widowed) show a 2.7 percent drop in live births between those with no education and those with one or two years, and a drop of 3.5 percent between the latter category and those with three or four.

[6] See *U.S. Census of Population, 1960: Puerto Rico*, PC (1) 53D, Table 95.

[7] It is of interest that even women with seven or eight years of education are having more than twice as many live births as the average Puerto Rican woman considers is the ideal number of children to have (two or less)—and only a fifth of the women get this far in school. See P. K. Hatt, *Backgrounds of Human Fertility in Puerto Rico* (Princeton: Princeton University Press, 1952), Table 37, p. 53.

As noted earlier, in evaluating or explaining the influence of education on fertility we must control other variables, probably the most important of which is residence. In Puerto Rico there is a marked relation between residence and education. For example, of legally married women aged 45 and over in 1960, 49 percent in San Juan, 59 percent in other urban areas, and 83 percent in rural areas have had less than five years of schooling.

In Table 77 we have introduced a three-category residential classification—the San Juan Standard Metropolitan Statistical Area, other urban areas, and rural areas.

Table 77. Total live births per 1,000 married women aged 45 and over, Puerto Rico, 1960 (legally married with spouses present), by education and residence

Years of school completed	San Juan SMSA	Urban	Rural
0	6,936	6,454	7,830
Primary			
1–4	5,962	5,865	7,626
5–6	5,078	4,942	6,886
7–8	3,924	4,106	5,271
Secondary			
1–3	3,032	3,295	4,454
4	2,386	2,525	2,648
College			
1 or more	1,909	1,938	1,931
Total	4,878	5,200	7,422

Source: See Table 76.

Although there is little difference between San Juan and other urban areas when education is controlled, both education and residence (rural and nonrural) show independent relationships with fertility. Over the total educational range—that is, from those with no education to those with one or more years of college—the rural areas show the greatest absolute and relative declines in fertility. Rural women of no education have had four times as many births as rural college women.

Urban fertility starts at a higher level that rural, but declines somewhat less over the entire educational range. The net effect is that toward the upper end of the educational range, differences in fertility by residence have virtually disappeared.[8] High educational inputs serve to equalize fertility at low levels among women of varying residence. The leveling out, however, does not occur until completion of high school.

An important question for the strategy of modernization relates to the timing and amounts of rural versus urban investments in education. In terms of effects on fertility, will the dollar invested in rural schools go as far as the dollar invested in urban schools?

Looking now at the degree of change in fertility associated with successive increments of education within each residential area (Table 78), we find that rural and urban areas have somewhat different patterns. The modest declines in fertility which

Table 78. Percentage change in fertility (live births per 1,000 legally married women, 45 and over) between successive educational categories, by residence, Puerto Rico, 1960

Between educational categories	San Juan SMSA and urban	Rural
o and 1–4	−11.5	−2.6
1–4 and 5–6	−15.2	−9.7
5–6 and 7–8	−20.1	−23.4
7–8 and 1–3 high school	−21.9	−15.5
1–3 and 4 high school	−22.4	−40.5
4 high school and college	−20.9	−27.1

Source: See Table 76.

[8] Jaffe found that urban and rural differences disappeared after ten years of education. Since part of the San Juan metropolitan area was classified as rural, he speculated that "a higher proportion of the better educated 'rural' women were residing in the metropolitan area and conforming to urban rather than rural ways of life." *Op. cit.,* p. 181.

we saw characteristic for the Commonwealth as a whole at the primary school level are *especially* characteristic of rural areas. Despite the fact that education eventually levels out fertility differences between urban and rural areas, the same increases in education do not have the same effect on fertility in rural and urban areas at the same time. Thus urban fertility drops by 25 percent between women with no education and women with five or six years, but by only 12 percent for rural women. It would appear that modest inputs of education have a negligible impact in rural areas, but a more important effect in urban areas. To summarize, a little education goes a longer way in the urban areas, but a lot of education goes farthest in rural areas.

If fertility is closely related to education, even when other variables are controlled, what accounts for this relation? While physiological and nutritional factors should not be ignored, there is good reason to believe that the major explanation lies in deliberate attempts by couples to limit their fertility. As obvious as this point may seem, it is sometimes seemingly denied by nondemographers who imply that education could be a *substitute* for birth control.

Table 79 shows data from a sample survey conducted in Puerto Rico in 1953, relating the practice of birth control to residence and education.

Table 79. Percent who have used a birth control method, by residence and education, Puerto Rico, 1953[a]

Education	Urban	Rural
0	40	26
1–4	40	35
5–8	57	37
9 or more	71	64

[a] While the sample was representative of the population of Puerto Rican households, the reported data for 767 couples refer to the married or consensually married population. See R. Hill, J. M. Stycos, and K. W. Back, *The Family and Population Control* (Chapel Hill: University of North Carolina Press, 1959), Table 78, p. 164.

Consistent with our findings on fertility we see that:

(1) Urban residence and years of education are independently and positively related to the practice of birth control.

(2) At the high school level, differences in contraceptive practice virtually disappear between urban and rural families.

(3) The largest impact of education on contraceptive practice occurs after elementary school, in both urban and rural areas. However, the data do not support the hypothesis that a little education has more impact in the urban areas.

DISCUSSION

An overall conclusion to be drawn from our varied analyses is that education possesses little of the magic character often attributed to it with respect to fertility. The fact that Latin American nations with the highest degree of education tend to have the lowest birth rates we found largely explicable in terms of their greater urbanization. Within countries, the clearest ecological relation between education and fertility occurs for the more developed nations, or for the more urbanized areas within nations.

Survey data for individual Peruvian women disclosed little differential fertility prior to the completion of primary school. Age at marriage helped to account for much of the differentials by education, but regional differences are more likely to be accounted for by contraceptive or abortive practices.

Recent census data from Puerto Rico show marked differential fertility by education. However, the fact that the differences *accelerate* with education, with major declines occurring only after elementary school is achieved, may account for the slow response of the birth rate, for much of Puerto Rico's educational gains have been at lower levels.

The implications for Latin American countries with currently high birth rates are not favorable. Puerto Rico's educational gains have been accomplished in a most propitious milieu for fertility decline, i.e., they have been accompanied by marked gains in per capita income, urbanization, and industrialization. (In 1950 its per capita commercial energy consumption was exceeded only by Argentina, Venezuela, and Chile; its per capita income only by Venezuela.) Thus, educational gains have not occurred in a "socioeconomic vacuum," as they may occur in some Latin American countries.

In any event, most Latin American countries are well behind Puerto Rico in education. In 1950 at least eleven Latin American countries showed higher illiteracy rates than did Puerto Rico in *1930;* and the average level of schooling in most Latin countries is well below the point where crucial drops in fertility were seen to take place in Puerto Rico. In 1950, in at least nine Latin countries, more than three-quarters of the males aged 25 and over had completed less than four years of primary school, and in only two countries and Puerto Rico was this figure under 50 percent.[9] For the sixteen Latin American countries where data were available, only about 7 percent of the total population aged 15 years and over had more than six years of education. The average years completed in these countries were 2.2, as opposed to 4.5 in Puerto Rico.[10] Most striking of all are data from the mid-fifties which indicate that only about one in every four or five who began school in Latin America ever completed the elementary level, and only one in twenty completed secondary school.[11] Given the facts that educational levels are generally low, that urbanization may be needed to activate the effect of education on fertility, and that Latin America is predominantly rural, Latin American countries which wait for "education" to reduce birth rates may wait a long time.

[9] *United Nations Compendium of Social Statistics: 1963,* Table 60.

[10] See O. Vera, "The Educational Situation and Requirements in Latin America," *op. cit.,* Table 3.

[11] *Ibid.,* pp. 291, 303.

17

Urbanization and Fertility
in Latin America

Much has been made of Latin America's rapid urbanization as a forerunner of declining fertility. It is true that with a quarter of its population residing in places of 20,000 or more in 1950, Latin America's level of urbanization compares favorably with such countries as Greece, Hungary, or Lebanon. However, the recency of this extensive urbanization is often overlooked. Around the start of the century "the only countries with more than 10 percent of their total population in cities of 20,000 or more were Argentina, Chile, Uruguay, and Cuba."[1] Venezuela, which by 1950 had a third of its population in cities, had only 7 percent in 1920, and 17 percent in 1936. Secondly, we must not neglect the fact that most countries are still primarily agricultural. As late as 1950, only five nations had less than half their active population engaged in agriculture. Finally, urbanization is of a particular kind in Latin America, one in which heavy concentrations of power, people, and culture occur in one city or very few cities,[2] where service occupations predominate along

[1] H. L. Browning, "Recent Trends in Latin American Urbanization," *Annals of the American Academy of Political and Social Science,* CCCXVI (March 1958), 111.

[2] One evidence of this is the high primacy pattern. "No other world region displays so consistently the pattern in which the primary or first city is many times larger than the second city . . . in 16 countries the first city is at least 3.7 times larger than the second city," and in 8 countries at least 7 times larger. Browning, *op. cit.,* 114–15.

with a minimum of factory manufacturing, and where the gulf between urban and rural is especially marked. All of this raises important questions concerning the degree and nature of urban-rural fertility differentials, and whether or when urban patterns may be expected to diffuse to rural areas.

Is there a significant rural-urban fertility differential? Although one has long been assumed for Latin America, the recent work of Robinson raised serious questions about basing such a belief on child-woman ratios.[3] Further, a recent U.N. analysis, while concluding that "in this region the fertility of the urban population is uniformly below that of the total population," also concluded that "the most striking feature of the data is the absence of any systematic relationship between degree of urbanization and level of fertility."[4] Because of the importance of this basic question, it will be necessary to review the evidence for a relationship, both among and within nations.

At the most general level, a strong relation is apparent between a nation's degree of urbanization and its level of fertility. To establish this we ran correlations between various measures of fertility and various measures of urbanization and economic development for nineteen Latin American countries and Puerto Rico (Table 80).

All the urbanization measures are correlated negatively with all of the fertility measures. Of the latter, however, the crude birth rate showed the highest correlations with urbanization, while percent in places 20,000 and over and percent in places 100,000 and over correlated more highly with fertility than do either percent in places 5,000 and over or percent in metropolitan areas. The former urbanization measures show higher corre-

[3] W. C. Robinson, "Urbanization and Fertility: The Non-Western Experience," *Milbank Memorial Fund Quarterly*, XLI (July 1963).

[4] Population Branch, United Nations, "Demographic Aspects of Urbanization in Latin America" in P. M. Hauser, ed., *Urbanization in Latin America* (New York: International Documents Service, 1961), pp. 103–04. Unfortunately, documentation for both statements was deleted from the published report.

Table 80. Correlation coefficients for measures of fertility, urbanization, and economic development, 20 Latin American countries around 1950 (Uruguay excluded)

Urbanization and development measures	Child-woman ratio[a]	Crude birth rate[a]	General fertility rate[a]	Total fertility rate[a]
Percent in places 5,000 +[b]	-.59	-.77	-.72	-.69
Percent in places 20,000 +[c]	-.65	-.80	-.76	-.72
Percent in places 100,000 +[c]	-.66	-.83	-.78	-.72
Percent in metropolitan areas 100,000 +[b]	-.41	-.72	-.65	-.65
Percent of population 15 years and older illiterate[d]	.33	.61	.52	.48
Percent of population 5–14 years enrolled in secondary schools[d]	-.41	-.70	-.63	-.60
Per capita gross national product[e]	.07	-.26	-.16	-.19
Percent of population 15–44 years in agriculture[f]	.49	.74	.66	.61

Sources:

[a] Lee Jay Cho, "Estimated Refined Measures of Fertility for all Major Countries of the World," *Demography*, I, No. 1 (1964). For those countries requiring estimates, Cho employed the equations prepared by D. J. Bogue and J. A. Palmore, "Some Empirical and Analytic Relations Among Demographic Fertility Measures, with Regressive Models for Fertility Estimation," *ibid.*

[b] Harley Browning, "Recent Trends in Latin American Urbanization," *Annals of the American Academy of Political and Social Science*, CCCXVI (March 1958).

[c] Philip M. Hauser, ed., *Urbanization in Latin America* (New York: International Documents Service, 1961), p. 94.

[d] Oscar Vera, "The Educational Situation and Requirements in Latin America," in *Social Aspects of Economic Development in Latin America*, Vol. I, Egbert DeVries and José Echaverría, eds. (UNESCO, 1963). Mexican and Peruvian figures were obtained from UNESCO, *World Illiteracy at Mid Century* (Geneva, 1957).

[e] Drawn mainly from The Research Center in Economic Development and Cultural Change of the University of Chicago, *The Role of Foreign Aid in the Development of Other Countries* (Washington: U.S. Government Printing Office, 1957); see also Norton Ginsberg, *Atlas of Economic Development* (Chicago: University of Chicago Press, 1961), p. 18.

[f] Drawn mainly from Food and Agriculture Organization of the United Nations, *Production Yearbook, 1958* (Rome, 1959); see also Ginsberg, *op. cit.*, p. 32.

lations with fertility than do the measures of education, per capita product or percent in agriculture. (All correlations are lowered when confined to the twelve countries where either vital statistics or census data are considered deficient. Thus, the correlations between percent in places 20,000 and over with the fertility measures are −.41, −.58, −.49, and −.42; for the remaining eight countries the comparable correlations are −.82, −.93, −.93, and −.92).

At the next level, we can relate fertility to the urban characteristics of subunits within countries. Child-woman ratios and other social characteristics were computed at the International Population Program for the smallest administrative unit (province, municipio, or department) reported in the 1950 censuses of eleven Latin American countries, a total of 312 units.[5] In only two countries, Venezuela and Honduras, does the correlation between child-woman ratio and urbanization (by each nation's definition) fall below −.50. The mean correlation for the eleven countries is −.66.[6] The correlations with urbanization are usually somewhat higher than with literacy or with percent in agriculture (Table 81).

[5] Despite a priori limitations of the child-woman ratio as a measure of fertility, it would appear to bear a close relation to more direct measures. For 8 Latin American countries with both good census and vital statistics data (Argentina, Chile, Costa Rica, Guatemala, Mexico, Panama, El Salvador, and Puerto Rico), the correlations between the child-woman ratio and the birth rate, general fertility rate and total fertility rate are .84, .92, and .91 respectively. (Bogue and Palmore report correlations of .93, .96, and .96 for 50 countries with good data.) Data for 22 Peruvian departments in 1940 show a correlation of .70 between child-woman ratios and births per 100 women 45+. See Chapter 14.

[6] Davis reports correlation coefficients for several other countries: Brazil −.80, Cuba −.92, Dominican Republic −.77, Ecuador −.50, Haiti −.71, and Peru −.56. The correlations for Argentina, Costa Rica and Panama reported in his series are considerably higher than ours, possibly because fewer units were employed. An average correlation of −.70 was found for 16 countries. K. Davis, "The Place of Latin America in World Demographic History," *Milbank Memorial Fund Quarterly*, XLII (April 1964), p. 47.

Table 81. Correlations between child-woman ratio and percent urban
for administrative subunits of 11 countries, around 1950

Country	Correlation coefficient	Number of units
Argentina	−.57	24
Bolivia	−.61	9
Chile	−.71	25
Costa Rica	−.72	65
El Salvador	−.88	14
Guatemala	−.70	22
Honduras	−.17	16
Mexico	−.60	32
Nicaragua	−.73	17
Panama	−.63	64
Venezuela	−.38	23

Source: Basic data from material censuses. Child-woman ratios refer
to children 0–4 per 100 women 15–44. "Urban" as defined by each national census.

While inferences drawn from ecological data employing a
crude fertility measure are risky, more direct and refined data
for selected Latin American countries show quite conclusively
that urban fertility is substantially lower than rural. For Cuba
and Panama the urban gross reproductive rates are half the rural,
in Puerto Rico and Brazil about two-thirds, and in Mexico three-
quarters.[7] Similar data for other countries are needed, but on
the whole the available data all point to a negative relation between fertility and urbanization. I believe that the highest research priority concerns the explanation of this relationship. A
few relevant questions and hypotheses are discussed below.

(1) To what extent is the magnitude of the rural-urban differential related to the degree and kind of urbanization? A U.N.
analysis concludes that "the figures available suggest that relative
differences between urban and rural fertility are apparently un-

[7] R. O. Carleton, "Fertility Trends and Differentials in Latin America,"
Milbank Memorial Fund Annual Quarterly, XLIII (October 1965).

related to the degree of urbanization within the country."[8] Further, the degree of correlation between urbanization and child-woman ratios within the subunits of a nation bears only a small relation to the degree of urbanization of the nation as a whole. The correlations between the former coefficients and percent in places of over 5,000, 20,000, 100,000 and metropolitan areas of over 100,000 are only .18, .32 and .42 respectively.[9] On the other hand, analyses of data for thirteen countries show a correlation of .60 between the ratio of rural to urban fertility ratios and percent in places of 20,000 and over. (Correlation with other urban measures varies from .52 to .56.) The question would appear still to be open.

(2) What is the nature of the lower urban fertility levels? Here I refer to the necessity for basic work on the components of differentials reflected in crude birth rates or child-woman ratios. Carleton has shown the urban-rural differentials as reflected by these measures are *increased* when gross reproduction rates are utilized (at least in five countries), suggesting that peculiarities of age and sex structure are not responsible for the differentials.[10]

In addition, we should learn the extent to which the residential variations are based on differential rates of motherhood or of the fertility of mothers. An illustration can be provided from calculations derived from the 1950 censuses of Panama and Mexico, where urban-rural differentials in births per woman are considerably reduced as one moves from births per woman to births per mother. In Panama, the proportion of women who are mothers in the 15–19 age group is almost twice as high in rural as in urban areas, and in the 20–24 age category a third

[8] Population Branch, United Nations, "Demographic Aspects of Urbanization in Latin America," *op. cit.*, p. 103.

[9] For the correlation coefficients between child-woman ratios and percent urban for subunits within nations, we used data reported by K. Davis for 17 countries. See "The Place of Latin America in World Demographic History," *op. cit.*

[10] Carleton, *op. cit.*

higher. For these age groups the urban-rural differential is virtually accounted for by the difference in the incidence of motherhood (Table 82).

Table 82. Index numbers for children ever born, rural areas, Panama and Mexico, 1950, by age (urban rate = 100)

Age	Panama		Mexico	
	All women	Mothers only	All women	Mothers only
15–19	211	107	200	107
20–24	162	120	144	120
25–29	160	138	155	139
30–34	174	154	137	123
35–39	184	161	139	129
40–44	180	156	126	117
45–49	168	148	127	118

Source: National censuses. In the case of Mexico "urban" refers to the Distrito Federal, "rural" to the remainder of the nation.

This phenomenon was even more marked in the 1940 census of Peru, where differences of about 25 percent in live births per woman between Lima and the rest of Peru virtually disappear when live births per mother are considered. Most striking was the fact that for the 23 departments various social measures (urbanization, literacy, language) showed positive relations to births per mother, weak or no relations to births per woman, and negative relationships with proportion ever giving birth.[11] Clearly, similar analyses are needed for all countries.[12]

(3) *How* is urbanization related to fertility? In most cities of Latin America the level of income, education, female labor

[11] See Chapter 14.
[12] Results at a crude level are consistent with our findings: "With the exception of Argentina and Cuba, the ratio of urban to national fertility is higher for non-single women than for total women." Population Branch, "Demographic Aspects of Urbanization in Latin America," *op. cit.*, p. 104.

force participation, and church attendance, to name only a few variables, are much higher than in rural areas. To what extent are these variables, rather than "urbanization," responsible for the differential fertility? Or to put the question another way, if such variables are held constant, is there any variance left in fertility which might be ascribed to something called urbanization?

EDUCATION

At the international level we recall the crude birth rate showed correlations of —.80 with proportions living in places of 20,000 and over, —.70 with secondary school attendance, and .61 with illiteracy. The correlation between urbanization and the birth rate drops only to —.65 when illiteracy is held constant by partial correlation, and to —.60, —.80, and —.67 when secondary school attendance, per capita GNP and percent in agriculture are held constant, in turn. On the other hand, the correlation between the birth rate and secondary school attendance (—.70) is reduced to —.34 when urbanization is held constant; and the correlation between child-woman ratios and illiteracy (.32) becomes negative when urbanization is held constant (—.37).

Similarly, partials can be computed for intracountry comparison. In this instance national census definitions of "urban" are employed and education is measured by percent literate (Table 83).

Two types of countries emerge. Holding literacy constant does not materially weaken the relations between urbanization and fertility in Argentina, Costa Rica, and, to a lesser extent, Chile, El Salvador, and Venezuela, but obliterates it in the remaining countries, most of which are Central American.

Simultaneous controls on several crucial variables are possible in the case of Puerto Rico, where special tabulations related

Table 83. Partial correlations between child-woman ratios and percent urban holding constant percent of women single and percent literate, administrative subunits of 11 countries, around 1950

Country	Simple correlation	Holding literacy constant	Holding percent single constant
Argentina	−.57	−.74	.76
Bolivia	−.61	.40	.43
Chile	−.71	−.46	.09
Costa Rica	−.72	−.68	−.55
El Salvador	−.94	−.93	−.62
Guatemala	−.70	.03	−.26
Honduras	−.17	.07	.01
Mexico	−.60	.28	−.21
Nicaragua	−.73	.17	−.15
Panama	−.63	.27	−.085
Venezuela	−.38	−.36	.23

cumulative fertility rates to age, marital status, residence, education, and female employment (Table 84).

Despite the many controls, in 13 out of 14 comparisons rural fertility is higher than urban, suggesting that the urban influence is something over and above education, labor force status, and marital status. Of course, the character of each of these variables can be expected to vary from urban to rural, and the source of the differentials might lie here. When we keep in mind that urban women tend toward the upper educational levels and are more likely to be employed, the full impact of "urbanization" can be seen to be quite strong. Thus the illiterate rural housewife has almost *five times* as many children as the college-educated urban employee.

Similar tables for other nations are needed to determine whether the Puerto Rican pattern is common or unusual. Each of the variables associated with urbanization and fertility needs careful attention in its own right.

Table 84. Total live births per 1,000 legally married women aged 45 and over, by education, residence, and labor force status, Puerto Rico, 1960

Years of school completed	In labor force			Not in labor force		
	Urban	Rural	% Difference	Urban	Rural	% Difference
0	5,409	7,438	27	6,774	7,846	14
Primary						
1-4	5,062	7,040	28	6,020	7,571	22
5-6	4,413	6,193	29	5,098	6,981	27
7-8	3,500	4,101	17	4,105	5,493	25
Secondary						
1-3	2,382	3,711	36	3,342	4,680	29
4	2,266	2,517	11	2,505	2,710	8
University						
1+	1,668	1,784	7	2,516	2,080	-4

Source: Special tabulations, Census 1960.

EDUCATION AND SOCIAL CLASS

From Table 84 it is apparent that urban-rural fertility differentials in Puerto Rico tend to disappear as education increases, and that small amounts of education seem to have a greater "effect" in urban areas.[13] Our survey data from several types of communities in Peru indicated that the fertility of Lima women is lower than that of women from selected smaller communities, at all educational levels. Further, it is clear that education is *not* related to fertility in the small, more rural communities studied. However, variation in fertility by social class was strong within all communities studied.[14]

[13] For more detailed discussion of educational influences, see Chapter 16.

[14] From unpublished data, International Population Program.

In a similar survey in the city of Santiago, fertility drops by about half between educational extremes, but income here too appears to discriminate fertility levels more sharply.[15]

FEMALE EMPLOYMENT

On a world-wide level, Collver and Langlois found a correlation of —.60 between female employment and fertility for twenty countries.[16] The Puerto Rican data contained in Table 84 would also suggest a strong negative relation. An ecological analysis of the twenty-one nonmetropolitan departments of Peru showed that in 1940 completed fertility showed a fairly high negative correlation with female employment.[17] On the other hand, survey data for Lima (as well as comparable data for urban and rural Turkey), suggest no consistent differences in fertility or in attitudes toward family size and birth control between employed and nonemployed wives.[18] Based on sample survey data in Jamaica, Stycos and Back conclude: "We do not believe that employment status is causally related to fertility, but that fertility affects employment status, in the case of the more stable unions. Marital status, on the other hand, affects employment status both directly and through the medium of children."[19] Clearly, this is a high priority area for research, and

[15] L. Tabah and R. Samuel, "Preliminary Findings of a Survey on Fertility and Attitudes Toward Family Formation in Santiago, Chile," in C. V. Kiser, ed., *Research in Family Planning* (Princeton: Princeton University Press, 1962). Table 8.

[16] A. Collver and E. Langlois, "The Female Labor Force in Metropolitan Areas: An International Comparison," *Economic Development and Cultural Change*, X (July 1962), 384.

[17] D. M. Heer, "Fertility Differences between Indian and Spanish-Speaking Parts of Andean Countries," *Population Studies*, XVIII (July 1964).

[18] J. M. Stycos and R. Weller, "Female Working Roles and Fertility," *Demography*, IV, No. 1 (1967). Neither study distinguishes type of employment.

[19] J. M. Stycos and K. W. Back, *The Control of Human Fertility in Jamaica* (Ithaca, N.Y.: Cornell University Press, 1964), p. 183.

one which requires special techniques, such as longitudinal designs, to determine the direction and nature of a possible causal relation.

MARITAL STATUS

Since the proportion childless in urban areas seems to account for much of the urban-rural fertility differential, we might expect higher proportions of the urban population to be single. Since 1950, most countries have removed consensual unions from the single category, and it is possible to examine rural-urban differentials for a few Central American nations (Table 85).

Table 85. Index number for percent of urban women single, by age, 1950 (rural area = 100)

Age	El Salvador	Costa Rica	Panama	Guatemala	Guatemala (Urban *ladinas* vs. rural *indigenas*)
15–19	110	111	114	132	147
20–24	131	137	133	178	226
25–29	144	160	136	200	184
30–34	155	167	126	186	242
35–39	160	173	128	208	280
40–44	162	186	124	200	264

Source: National censuses. Urban-rural as defined by national censuses except Panama where Panama Province was compared with the rest of the country.

In each case urban women at all ages are more likely to be single, and there is a tendency for the discrepancy to increase with age, within the range presented. Most striking are the differences in Guatemala between urban *ladina* women and rural *indigenas*. At the upper ages there are close to three times as high a proportion single in the former as in the latter category.

The promising nature of this variable in accounting for urban-rural differentials is indicated in Table 83. When percent single is held constant by partial correlation, the originally high negative correlations between percent urban and child-woman ratios either disappears or becomes positive in 9 out of the 11 countries analyzed.

One consideration is that women separated from consensual unions are probably classified as single, and there may be considerable gross migration between the categories of single and consensual. The significance of these categories for fertility has been amply demonstrated for parts of the English-speaking Caribbean, and remains to be done for Latin America.

MIGRATION

A recent analysis of Puerto Rican data shows that women migrants have consistently lower fertility than nonmigrants, even when residence, age, marital status, education and employment status are controlled.[20] Migrant women in Jamaica also had lower fertility, especially if their marital status was "visiting" rather than common law married.[21] Again, the need for longitudinal studies is apparent, although much more can be done with retrospective histories of fertility and spatial and social mobility. In such studies, place-of-origin research should receive as much attention as place-of-destination.

BIOLOGICAL FACTORS

In an effort to account for marked urban-rural differentials in Jamaica, Stycos and Back covered the following variables in a sample survey: age, marital status, number of unions, length

[20] G. C. Myers and E. W. Morris, "Migration and Fertility in Puerto Rico," *Population Studies*, XX (July 1966).
[21] Stycos and Back, *op. cit.*, pp. 183–84.

of union, pattern of union, use of birth control, frequency of sexual relations, employment of females, and migration. Neither singly nor in combination could these variables "explain away" the rural-urban differentials. In noting the high degree of childlessness in the urban area, the authors speculate that venereal disease may be an important, though unexplored variable.[22] Although it can hardly be said that sufficient work has been done on demographic and social variables, our inability thus far to account for residential variations in fertility plus the almost total neglect of biological factors argue for assigning a fairly high priority to research in the latter area.

Studies on other regions suggest a relation between socioeconomic status (and therefore presumably better health) and early resumption of postpartum menstruation, higher age at menopause and fewer miscarriages. Furthermore, with respect to nutrition, although de Castro's thesis on the negative relation between protein intake and fertility has been generally discredited by demographers, we should avoid throwing out the baby with the bath. Of course, since better nutrition and health are more characteristic of urban areas, it is unlikely that these will explain inferior urban fertility. Indeed, specific fertility-depressing diseases aside, holding most health factors constant would probably magnify urban-rural differences.

FUTURE TRENDS IN FERTILITY

Even though the nature of the relation between fertility and urbanization is obscure, it might be thought that the fact of the relation is sufficient to predict imminent declines in fertility. Even this degree of optimism is unwarranted, however, for it is based on the assumption that national fertility rates will be substantially altered by the increasing proportions living in urban areas, and/or that urban patterns will diffuse to rural areas. With respect to the first assumption, Carleton's important analysis

[22] *Ibid.,* pp. 184–87.

shows that the effect of urban rates on national birth rates is minimal and that the continuing increase in proportions living in urban places probably will not, as such, have much impact on national rates.[23]

Concerning the diffusion hypothesis, there is reason to believe that there are greater barriers to the spread of urban ideas in Latin America than in other countries. Ethnic geographic obstacles in some nations, and traditional class and cultural barriers in others, imply that diffusion may be much slower than was presumably the case in European or North American nations. Thus, in Central American countries in 1950, the proportion of illiterates in rural areas ranged from two to six times as high as in urban areas.[24] These are gulfs difficult to bridge—even with modern mass media.

Argentina, usually cited as a promising example, has aspects which may make it unique. Its national birth rates have apparently been declining from the end of the nineteenth century, and it is not altogether clear whether urban declines preceded or were paralleled by rural fertility declines,[25] as was probably the case throughout the nineteenth century in the United States.[26] But general rural-urban disparities have probably been

[23] Carleton, *op. cit.*

[24] Drawn from data in *Human Resources of Central America, Panama and Mexico, 1950–1980*, ECLA Catalog No. 60, XIII.1, 1960, Table 18.

[25] Since no relation was found between child-woman ratios and urbanization for Argentina provinces up to 1914, but a strong relation was apparent in 1947, Davis concludes that "the limitation of birth apparently began in the cities." However, the absence of a relation in the earlier periods could also occur if rural and urban rates were both declining from similar high levels. See Davis, "The Place of Latin America in World Demographic History," *op. cit.*, p. 33.

[26] "After 1810 the declines in fertility ratios of the rural population more than kept pace with those of the urban population . . . declines in rural fertility had more effect on changes in national fertility than did the combined effect of (a) the increasing proportion of population residing in urban areas and (b) declines in urban fertility." W. H. Grabill, C. V. Kiser, and P. K. Whelpton, *The Fertility of American Women* (New York: John Wiley, 1958), pp. 16–17.

less in Argentina than in most Latin American countries, and the extent to which Argentina's history is relevant is not yet clear. It is still possible in places such as Argentina to contrast the fertility of first, second, and third generation Europeans. Longitudinal and cohort studies would be especially valuable here, but the whole question of the influence of the foreign born on the fertility of Latin American cities has been unexplored.

On the other hand, there are various factors which may keep Latin American fertility high or increasing. Better health and nutrition, increasing average length of reproductive span, reduced maternal mortality, more stable marital patterns, lowered age at marriage, and so on, are all factors which would be expected to increase fertility. Indeed, between 1950 and 1960 seven Latin American countries showed increases in general fertility rates in the order of 8 to 13 percent, while Panamanian rates increased by a fifth, and Jamaican by 40 percent. Only Argentina and Puerto Rico showed declines in this period.[27] Improved statistical services can only partially account for such increases.

Possibly these are short-run fluctuations, or they may be indications of the improving social and economic conditions which will eventually lead to a decline. Of course, the crucial question is: how long is "eventual"? If K. Davis's theory of "multiphasic response" is applicable to Latin America, it may not be "too" long.[28] What can we draw from this theory?

In examining historic demographic trends in Japan and in European nations, Davis finds that under certain conditions prolonged high rates of population increase lead to responses on the individual family level which result in slowing the rate of increase. Different societies emphasize different means—abortions,

[27] See J. C. Ridley, "Recent Natality Trends in Underdeveloped Countries," in M. C. Sheps and J. C. Ridley (Eds.) *Public Health and Population Change* (Pittsburgh: University of Pittsburgh Press, 1965).

[28] See K. Davis, "The Theory of Change and Reform in Modern Demographic History," *Population Index*, XXIX (October 1936); and "Population," *Scientific American*, CCIX (September 1963).

contraception, delayed marriage, emigration—but they all re-act. The reaction is due to "new opportunities on the one hand and larger families on the other."[29] Thus, a condition for the response to increased family size is a "fear of invidious depriva-tion" which is more likely to emerge when opportunities are present as a result of an expanding economy. What do we need to know about Latin American countries to be able to apply the theory?

Recent attention to Latin America's population explosion tends to obscure the important fact of the recency of rapid growth. The region as a whole has grown rapidly only in the past few decades, and in some countries much of the earlier growth was due to immigration rather than to natural increase. Despite the fact that mortality declines began in Latin America before they did in most of Asia and Africa, the most substantial declines are of relative recency. Thus, between the late 1930's and the late 1950's the registered death rate of one Central American country fell by a quarter, that of two others by a third, and in three declined by 40 to 50 percent.[30]

Given the recency of change in mortality, it may be that a perceptible increase in family size may only just be occurring in some countries, have occurred some time ago in others, and not have begun in still others. Determining when a "perceptible in-crease" in family size occurs is a complex matter requiring a combination of demographic, historical, and social psychologi-cal techniques. Clearly, we should first seek earlier data on rates of growth and the components of this growth, correcting what Davis calls the "tendency of analysts and commentators to evade historical study of Latin American demography."[31]

Second, we should recognize household size and family size

[29] Davis, "Population," *op. cit.*, p. 64.

[30] Computed from data in H. L. Geisert, *Population Problems in Mexico and Central America* (George Washington University, 1959), Table 5.

[31] Davis, "The Place of Latin America in World Demographic His-tory," *op. cit.*, p. 28.

as variables in their own right, variables which could influence and be influenced by fertility.

Third, for future data collection, we should introduce more questions in our surveys concerning perceptions of change in mortality, fertility, family size, and household size. This is not to say that an awareness of increased family size is necessary for a feeling of population pressure within the family; but where mortality declines as abruptly as it has in some Latin American countries, it is entirely plausible to expect an awareness of the change, and that awareness might precipitate a sense of population pressure. When such questions were recently introduced in a survey in Peru, it was found that the higher the social class the greater the perception of declines in both fertility and mortality. Unfortunately, the question of change in family household size was not asked, and the explanation for lower-class attitudes is therefore incomplete, since those who reported increasing fertility might be reflecting a perceived increase in household size. An interesting question for applied research would be the impact on motivation for family planning of the introduction of concrete information on increased family size. Finally, we need more data on the concept of "invidious deprivation." There is evidence from some countries that the urban lower classes desire fewer children than the upper classes, and this is due to an awareness of the high economic costs of children to families of low income. But we do not know the condition under which such attitudes are generated, their distribution in rural areas, nor the point at which they are translated into behavior.

CONCLUSION

Since knowledge of the causes and consequences of differential fertility in Latin America is rudimentary, it is suggested that the area of urbanization and fertility provide a broad research focus for investigation in the next decade. Research on urbanization lends itself particularly well to a blend of macro- and micro-sociology. In the former category, the relation of types of cities, degrees of urbanization, and trends in urbanization to fertility are particularly important; while sample surveys can profitably concentrate on the ways in which city life influences the constellation of attitudes toward mortality, family size, household size, aspiration level, and family planning. In between these levels much more needs to be known about the structure of rural-urban fertility variations—for example, the relative contributions of childlessness, subfecundity, sex ratio imbalances, and marital status. Studies of special groups—migrants and working women in particular—are of special importance, especially if longitudinal designs can be carried out. In the next decade cities will continue to grow in Latin America, and Latin Americans' interest in urbanization will grow even faster. The study of urbanization and fertility would not only be scientifically rewarding but would be assured of the public attention the topic deserves.

IV

CONCLUSIONS

18

The Prospects for Fertility
Control in Latin America

In the second half of the twentieth century, mankind has seen that for the first time in history rather precise control over both mortality and fertility was technologically feasible. Improved public health procedures, breakthroughs in contraceptive technology, and advancements in mass education techniques have brought the systematic control of human natural increase within reach. Continuing declines in mortality in Latin America suggest that one component of natural increase continues to be controlled; but there is little evidence of comparable changes in fertility. With the exceptions of Argentina, Chile, and, probably Uruguay, no Latin American nation has shown signs of a consistent decline in birth rates, although several have shown recent signs of increase.[1] Is Latin America doomed to perpetually high rates of natural increase?

Since the present rates of increase could not be maintained for very long without increases in mortality, the real questions become not whether, but when and how. Essentially, we must answer two prior questions: Are the people ready? and, Will governments act?

[1] For estimates of general fertility rates in earlier decades see K. Davis, "The Place of Latin America in World Demographic History," *Milbank Memorial Fund Quarterly*, XLII (April 1964).

POPULAR CONCERN FOR
POPULATION CONTROL

The first error that we should correct is the notion that nothing will happen if the state does not act; for in the face of current high rates of population increase and modest increases in per capita well-being, the people will act if the state will not. However, while acting in ways to relieve their sense of population pressure, they will create other social and economic problems which may be of equal magnitude. Let us review the ways in which societies respond to the threat of population growth, and assess the implications for Latin America.

Age at Marriage

One of the principal ways in which European countries traditionally kept fertility lower than the biological maximum was by delayed marriage. In modern times, Ireland has maintained low birth rates principally by delayed marriage and by nonmarriage. Since Latin America, like Ireland, is predominantly Roman Catholic, it might be thought that similar solutions could be achieved. There seems to be little similarity in marriage habits, however. In Ireland, less than one in every five women aged 20–24 has been married, but in Latin American countries, with the exception of Argentina and Chile (about 40 percent), over half of the women have already been married by this age.

Of course, there are predictable differences by social class. In the survey of Lima women discussed earlier, the mean age at first union was 22.4 for the highest of four social classes, and 19.1 for the lowest. This might suggest that as education and economic development increase, later ages at marriage will follow. However, there is a basic characteristic of marriage patterns in Latin America which makes such prediction hazardous: unlike Ireland, where despite the large number of unmarried people there is little illegitimacy and few consensual unions, in Latin America consensual unions and illegitimacy are widespread. On the one hand, if urbanization and economic development produce shifts from consensual to legal unions, fertility could be affected positively, if the West Indian situation, described earlier, prevails.[2] On the other hand, economic and population pressures might produce a decline in legal marriages and a corresponding increase in *de facto* unions and illegitimacy. Even if these should result in lower birth rates, one must ask whether it is worth the price of increased family instability.

Migration

A second, and perhaps the more traditional response to population pressure, is a redistribution of the population. Since the contemporary world leaves little opportunity for international redistribution of population, virtually all of the migratory response to population pressure now occurs intranationally. While this process is going on at a tremendous rate in Latin America, it is less effective as a solution to population pressures than has been the case in other regions and times. On the one hand, the rates of natural increase in Latin American countries far exceed any experienced by European countries, and, on the other, there are only limited possibilities for international migration. Further, the areas which least need population are the areas which are growing the fastest—the cities. It may be that in the long run such urbanization is to the benefit of the nations; but in the short run its excessive speed causes problems ranging from increased crime rates to urban political unrest. This would be a high price to pay even if the population problem were being solved. But there are additional reasons why the migration depending on private initiative is falling short of this effect. First, despite the massive exodus from rural areas, there are more people than ever before living in rural places, because of the very high birth rates. Indeed, in areas such as Haiti where there is also a shortage of land, the rural response to overpopulation has been severe fractionization of land

[2] J. M. Stycos and K. W. Back, *The Control of Human Fertility in Jamaica* (Ithaca, N.Y.: Cornell University Press, 1964); and J. Blake, *Family Structure in Jamaica* (Glencoe, Ill.: Free Press, 1961).

holdings, to the point of severely diminishing agricultural productivity. Second, urban fertility does not appear to be declining
at a significant rate, and as we have seen, there is little hope that
increasing urbanization will substantially alter national birth
rates.[3]

Postconception Controls

There probably has never been a society, past or present, in
which some method of limiting fertility was not practiced to
some extent. But in most societies, postconception controls—
infanticide and abortion—rather than contraception have been
practiced.

While the frequent utilization of infanticide in both preliter-
ate and classical western cultures is well known, it is less frequently realized that its use in the middle ages was so extensive
that it had to be singled out for special attention on the part of
church authorities. The frequency of infanticide in contemporary nations is unknown and we can only speculate that this
age-old method is still employed by desperate parents who know
no other way, or who begin their family planning too late.

Abortion is a method of equal antiquity but of much greater
significance in accounting for the birth levels of many contemporary nations. While we can only speculate on the impact
of abortion on the early fall of birth rates in France and other
North European nations, there is no doubt about its recent influence on societies as diverse as the Soviet Union and Japan.
These two nations perhaps show the fastest fertility declines on
record, the U.S.S.R.'s birth rate declining by a third in the
decade after 1925, Japan's by half in less than a decade in the
postwar period. In both instances national abortion programs
are often given the credit for the declines, but there is evidence
that the national programs only legalized and accelerated prac-

[3] See R. O. Carleton *"Fertility Trends and Differentials in Latin
America," Milbank Memorial Fund Quarterly*, XLIII (October 1965).

tices which were already widespread. Indeed, in both instances, the stamping out of clandestine abortions was a major justification for the initiation of the national programs.

In Latin America, physicians associated with the maternity services of hospitals have long been aware of the high incidence, because of the number of women hospitalized for complications due to induced abortion. The whole topic, however, was officially ignored. Diagnostic classifications in hospital records were often vague, the topic was rarely discussed at medical conferences, and each country tended to regard the problem as unique. A small bombshell was dropped in 1962, however, when Drs. Armijo and Monreal of Chile presented a paper on the epidemiology of abortion in Santiago to the Seventh Pan American Congress of Social Medicine.[4] Participants were startled to hear this problem discussed openly and frankly, and even more surprised to discover that other countries shared their "unique" problems.

The Armijo-Monreal paper was the first in a Chilean series based on household probability samples involving interviews with nearly 3,800 women aged 20–50 in the cities of Santiago, Concepción, and Antofagasta. The study disclosed a startling incidence—just under one out of every four women interviewed admitted at least one induced abortion, ranging from 15 percent in Concepción to 27 percent in Antofagasta. Of the aborting women, a quarter had already had three or more abortions.[5] It was also found that a third of the Santiago abortions resulted in hospitalization—ranging from over half of those performed by the women themselves, to less than a quarter of those performed by doctors or midwives.[6] These results were publicized around

[4] R. Armijo and T. Monreal, "Epidemiología del Aborto en Santiago," *Revista Médica Panamericana*, X (August 1963).

[5] R. Armijo and T. Monreal, "The Problem of Induced Abortion in Chile," *Milbank Memorial Fund Quarterly*, XLIII (October 1965).

[6] R. Armijo and T. Monreal, "Factores Asociados a las Complicaciones del Aborto Provocado," *Revista Chilena de Obstetricia y Ginecología*, XCI (April 1963).

the same time that other investigators were assessing the costs to the national health service of hospitalizing abortion cases. It was found that approximately 184,000 hospital "bed-days" were expended on abortion cases in a single year (1960); that 42 percent of the general admissions to emergency services were abortion cases; and that abortion represented over a third of the surgical treatments given in the obstetrical services of the hospitals surveyed.[7]

The addition of economic to the moral and health considerations produced even greater concern, and a number of investigations were initiated or announced in other countries. Preliminary results parallel the Chilean. Thus, in Buenos Aires intensive interviewing was carried out among the 600 female patients aged 35–49 who attended nonobstetrical or psychiatric clinics of the Guillermo Rawson Hospital in 1964. Over 25 percent of all pregnancies were found to have been terminated in induced abortions.[8] In a representative sample of households in Rio de Janeiro in 1963, of the 1,585 married or mated women aged 20–25 who had had at least one live birth, 10 percent had also had at least one induced abortion.[9] The lowest reported incidence thus far comes from Lima, where a survey was confined to younger women, aged 20–39. Less than 5 percent of the pregnancies of these women had resulted in an induced abortion, according to their own admission.[10] More impressive data

[7] S. Plaza and H. Briones, "Demanda de Recursos de Atención Médica del Aborto Complicado," Congreso Médico Social Panamericano, Santiago, Chile, 1962 (mimeo.).

[8] Nydia Gomes Ferrarotti and Carmen García Varela, "Investigaciones Sobre Incidencia del Aborto Criminal," unpublished paper, 1964; and "Encuesta Sobre el Aborto y sus Variables, Incluyendo Métodos de Planificación 'de Familia,'" *Revista de la Sociedad de Obstetricia y Ginecología de Buenos Aires*, No. 611 (December 1964).

[9] B. Hutchinson, "Induced Abortion in Brazilian Married Women," *América Latina*, VII (October-December, 1964).

[10] M. F. Hall, "Birth Control in Lima, Peru: Attitudes and Practices," *Milbank Memorial Fund Quarterly*, XLIII (October 1965).

have been reported for other countries, ranging from three provoked abortions for every live birth in Uruguay,[11] to 15 percent of all pregnancies in Guatemala.[12] Whatever the precise figures, there is little doubt that abortion rates in Latin American cities are higher than anyone suspected.

It should not be thought that the higher rates reported are primarily due to pregnancies stemming from promiscuous relations. The Brazilian incidence data are based only on married women, and over three-quarters of the Argentine abortions occurred to married women. In the Santiago study, 85 percent of the induced abortions occurred to married women, who constituted 71 percent of the entire sample.[13]

Not only is the incidence of induced abortion high, but there is evidence that the rate is *increasing*. Where there were eight hospitalized abortion cases per hundred live births in Chilean hospitals in 1937, there were nineteen by 1958.[14] In the Caracas maternity hospital Concepción Palacio, where there was one abortion for every twelve live births in 1939, there was one for every four in 1964.[15]

Under present conditions in Latin America, abortion is painful, dangerous, sinful, expensive, and illegal. The growing rates

[11] I. Rosada, "La Situación del Aborto Voluntario en el Uruguay, Posibles Soluciones," Fourth Conference of the Western Hemisphere Region, International Planned Parenthood Federation, San Juan, P.R., April 1964 (mimeo).

[12] Roberto Santiso, "Contraceptives as a Means of Combating Illegal Abortions," Fourth Conference of the International Planned Parenthood Federation, Western Hemisphere Region, San Juan, P.R., April 1964 (mimeo).

[13] R. Armijo and T. Monreal, "Epidemiología del Aborto provocado en Santiago," *op. cit.*, p. 38.

[14] T. Monreal, "El Aborto Provocado, Síntesis Bibliográfica Reciente," *Cuadernos Médico-Sociales* (Chile), II, No. 2 (1961).

[15] L. A. Angulo Arévalo, "Atitudes ante la Fecundidad en General y Particularmente en Venezuela," Congreso Venezolano de Salud Pública, March 1966 (mimeo).

indicate that the public, especially in urban areas, is taking matters into its own hands in the absence of public services for family planning. This is precisely what happened in Japan, the Soviet Union, and other East European countries prior to their legalization of abortion.

On the other hand, Latin American governments can anticipate a bloody battle with the Church should the legalization of abortion facilities be considered. This, plus the expensiveness of a method relative to contraceptive controls, are among the costs of such programs—but the costs to the society of high rates of illegal abortion are even greater.

Contraception

While contraceptive techniques have been known to societies from the ancient Egyptians to the contemporary Sumatra primitives, most of the methods have had serious drawbacks such as difficulty of application, low efficiency, and costliness. Consequently their use has tended to be restricted to upper-class groups or highly motivated individuals. Toward the latter part of the nineteenth century, however, a greater democratization of knowledge on birth control occurred in Europe, and use of the douche, coitus interruptus, and the condom became quite widespread. Clearly, modern levels of fertility were achieved *without* modern contraceptive technology. Could the same not be expected in Latin America?

Results from the CELADE surveys show interesting differences among cities, but on the whole confirm findings from earlier studies in the Caribbean, Peru, and Chile. Most women do not regard a large family as ideal, and if they could choose the number of children for themselves, would have three or four. Furthermore, the majority of the women have already tried some method of contraception.[16] (See Table 86.)

[16] C. Miró and F. Rath, "Preliminary Findings of Comparative Fertility Surveys in Three Latin American Countries," *Milbank Memorial Fund Quarterly*, XLIII (October 1965). Based on sales data, H. Levin estimates

Table 86. Preliminary data from CELADE sample surveys conducted among married women, 20–50, in six Latin American cities

City	Preferred number of children	Percent who have practiced contraception
Bogotá	3.6	40
Caracas	3.5	59
Mexico City	4.2	38
Panama City	3.5	60
Rio de Janeiro	2.7	58
San José	3.6	65

Although Rio de Janeiro seems somewhat unusual in terms of small family ideals, let us use this city as an example for more detailed analysis, since further data are available. The average woman interviewed had had only 2.3 live births at the time she was interviewed, but when asked if they wanted any more, eight out of every ten replied negatively. The differences by social class are especially interesting. Women with university training have the largest ideal family size (2.9) and those who have not gone beyond primary school the smallest (2.5). "Of women in the highest status category, 23.4 percent regarded one or two children as the ideal. On the other hand, as many as 42.6 percent of women in the lowest category wanted only this number of children."[17] However, class differences in fertility itself are exactly the reverse. Women with no education have had 3.3 births, those with some university training just over one. Thus, the lower classes, who want the fewest children, in fact have the most.

This same pattern of relationships was found in Peru, both in Lima and in the provincial city of Chimbote. It should also be recalled from Chapter 10 that the lower classes were much more

that in Argentina at least 350,000 women are using oral contraceptive pills, in Chile 67,000, and in Peru 55,000. Private Report, Population Council, 1966.

[17] Hutchinson, *op. cit.*, p. 32.

sensitive than the upper classes to the economic liabilities of ad-ditional children. Why then do the lower classes have more? Probably because they marry earlier, practice less contraception, and practice it less effectively. Perhaps, too, ignorance of mod-ern contraceptive techniques, and disenchantment or failure with methods such as coitus interruptus or rhythm may lead many women into abortion. In Rio de Janeiro, women who had aborted were more likely than others to have practiced contra-ception, and the lower the social class the more likely was this method to have been coitus interruptus, the safe period, or folk techniques. In the Buenos Aires study, about half the abortions had been preceded by contraceptive practice, and in 83 percent of these cases coitus interruptus was the method employed.[18] In Peru, although the incidence of overall contraceptive practice declined from about two-thirds of the upper-class women to just over a third of the lower class, the use of coitus interruptus and douche increased from 4 percent of the upper to 44 percent of the lower-class users.[19]

The spread of contraceptive knowledge to the rural and lower classes may be expected "eventually," but it is again a question of whether the time required to effect such changes "naturally" is worth the price. Such changes are usually the concomitant of broad social changes such as industrialization, education, and so-cial mobility, but these changes must be substantial before any major change in fertility is effected. In Puerto Rico, for exam-ple, we recall that women showed little variation in fertility prior to six years of education. Only in the heavily industrial-ized, urbanized, and well-educated nations of Argentina and Uruguay do we see modern fertility levels in Latin America. If other nations must await comparable development there will be enormous population increase in the interim.

[18] Armijo and Monreal found such a low incidence of *coitus interruptus* in Chile that the possibility of faulty interviewing techniques must be entertained.

[19] M. F. Hall, *op. cit.*, Table 2.

DEVELOPMENTS IN THE PUBLIC SECTOR

Although popular concern for family planning seems reasonably high, it does not follow that major impacts on the birth rate can soon be expected. The same studies which demonstrated positive motivation for family planning and relatively high incidence of its use also demonstrate great ignorance on the part of the public concerning the range of modern contraceptives available, as well as erratic patterns of contraceptive practice. In order to activate preferences for small families and precipitate effective and appropriate behavior toward these ends, both contraceptive information and supplies must become readily available to the public.

We have seen however, that the official positions of Latin American nations have been in opposition to any action in this sphere, and that many intellectuals have been indifferent to population problems. Further, there is restrictive legislation about the dissemination of contraception in large areas of Latin America, and the whole subject has been, in the words of Lleras Camargo, "the great tabu of our time."

In the light of these circumstances is there any hope for public programs of family planning in Latin America? Indeed there is, as a result of truly remarkable shifts in the climate of discussion and in the opinion of Latin American intellectuals—changes which only began to be apparent in the early 1960's. A number of factors account for the change.

The Shift from Private to Public Opinion

There is no doubt that toward the mid-1960's there was a very great increase in attention to population problems and, partly as a result of the Catholic Church's example, population problems and birth control ceased to be tabooed topics and became public currency.

In 1965, Cornell University's International Population Program began to collect and analyze Latin American newspaper articles dealing with population problems. Within two years, close to 15,000 articles were collected, almost two-thirds of them dealing with birth control. As a concrete example, between September 1965 and April 1967 a reader of the two leading Bogotá dailies (*El Tiempo* and *El Espectador*) was exposed to an article on population every other day, on the average. No European or North American reader had anything like this degree of exposure to information prior to or during the periods of national fertility decline.[20]

Availability of New Census Data

While the 1960's saw little improvement in data on births and deaths, there was a major innovation in census data for a number of countries—the provision of population trend data accurate enough to assess past and project future rates of population growth. The 1950 censuses of the Americas represented a technical breakthrough, with comparable definitions, standards, and procedures introduced in many countries for the first time. Thirteen of the countries which took censuses in 1950 took them again in 1960, yielding relatively reliable measures of decennial growth.

The results were startling, even to experts. As late as 1960 the Economic Commission for Latin America and the United Nations Demographic Center in Chile estimated the region's population at 210 million; but by 1962 it was evident that the populations were six and a half million larger than this.[21] This information was not only widely circulated in the press, but led to more detailed analyses of census data than had been characteristic for earlier censuses.

[20] See J. M. Stycos "Colombian Newspapers and the Birth Control Controversy" paper read to the 1967 meetings of the American Sociological Association (August 1967).

[21] C. Miró, "The Population of Latin America," *Demography*, I, No. 1 (1964).

The Emerging Importance of National Planning

As a result both of internal foment for reform and Alliance for Progress pressures for rational planning of social and economic reform, many Latin American countries have in recent years introduced national planning and national planning boards. Planning, whether for schools, roads, industrial development, or agrarian reform, forces the planners to face the implications of population growth, and makes them far more interested in demographic data than ever before. Moreover, since most countries of Latin America are feeling frustrated at the slow per capita economic and agricultural gains, there is a growing willingness to consider population growth as a variable, subject to rational planning, rather than a fact to which all other aspects of the economy must be adjusted.

Medical Concern over Abortion Rates

While economists are becoming increasingly alarmed over the implications of population growth for economic development, we have noted that the medical profession is becoming alarmed at the evidence provided by scientific studies of the increase of individual abortions. A number of pilot programs for the spread of contraceptive practices have been introduced in Latin America as abortion control programs, rather than as population control.

Public Sensibility to Urbanization

A population growth rate of 2 to 3 percent per year is of a magnitude which is not noticeable to the average citizen; but a growth rate of 5 to 10 percent probably is, especially when the growth is concentrated geographically or socially. Thus, while *national* growth of population may not be readily visible, the great postwar growth of Latin American cities is a striking phenomenon to all its citizens, especially its articulate ones. The middle and upper classes tend to be alarmed and fearful of the growing "bandas de miseria" which surround the cities with restive migrants. A sense of *population pressure* never before experienced by the elite has been created.

Availability of North American Funds and Technical Assistance

Most North American foundations, universities, and private and public organizations concerned with population problems began to operate in Latin America only within the past few years, as the combined result of two more general developments: the increased resources being devoted to population problems everywhere, and the increased attention to Latin American problems generally, after at least two decades of neglect.

Partly as a result of the efforts of Teodoro Moscoso, a veteran of Puerto Rico's struggles with population control, the Agency for International Development's Latin American Division was the most active geographic branch in promoting assistance on population problems to requesting nations. While only $209,500 was expended in 1965, over one and a half million dollars was expended by AID for population and family planning activities in 1966, and close to three million allocated for 1967. The Western Hemisphere branch of the International Planned Parenthood Federation moved from a grant budget of only $283,559 in 1965 to $1,163,245 in 1967, and more than doubled its staff. The Population Council, which averaged less than $200,000 per year in grants to Latin American institutions in 1962–1963, granted nearly $700,000 in 1965. The Ford Foundation, which granted only $260,000 in 1962, expended over one and a half million in 1966.

The foregoing tells us *why* a major shift in public opinion among intellectual circles in Latin America is occurring. We have still to examine the more concrete evidences of the shift, and the expected consequences for population control. The most significant developments have occurred only since 1964, and we will confine our discussion to this period.

Several significant steps were taken within the traditionally cautious inter-American system. In September of 1964 an unprecedented meeting was held at the Pan-American Union for Latin American ambassadors to the Organization of American States and to the United States. Organized largely as the result of efforts by William Draper and Alberto Lleras Camargo, the ambassadors were exposed to a concentrated dosage of discussion of Latin American population problems by a distinguished list of speakers. Soon thereafter the Inter-American Economic and Social Council recommended that "studies should be carried out to determine the requirements of economic development and social progress as they relate to population increase. . . . Consequently, IA-ECOSOC recommends that Latin American countries carry out such studies, and charges CIAP with coordinating them on an international level and with providing the countries necessary technical assistance."[22] As a result of this mandate, the Department of Social Affairs of the OAS General Secretariat proposed to the Inter-American Committee on the Alliance for Progress (CIAP) that the OAS Secretariat develop a program on population problems of Latin America. In April 1965, CIAP suggested that "governments carefully consider the need to formulate population policies and put them into effect . . . that they make . . . studies on mutual relation between population trends and factors of economic and social development . . . and problems relating to fertility and economic, political, and religious factors that condition it."[23] The Department of Social Affairs of the OAS was charged with coordinating these and other activities relating to population problems, and in 1967 sponsored a major conference on population problems of the hemisphere.

In October 1965, the Directing Council of the Pan American Health Organization voted to request the Director "to provide technical advice as requested on the health aspects of population

[22] OEA/SER. H/XIII, p. 41.
[23] Mimeographed letter from Theo R. Crevenna, Department of Social Affairs, OAS (May 19, 1965).

dynamics and . . . to cooperate with CIAP in (population) studies assigned to it."[24] In October of 1966 they voted the establishment of Regional Education and Research Training Centers on health aspects of population dynamics; and the establishment of an Office of Health and Population Dynamics, including a Population Information Center.

In the meantime, national governments and private agencies were even more active. While the first three conferences of the International Planned Parenthood Federation, Western Hemisphere Region, had barely been able to muster a bona fide Latin American delegate, the fourth conference, held in April 1964, attracted high-level participation from virtually all Latin countries, and official government delegates from twelve Latin American nations. The delegates approved a resolution calling on the OAS, the Pan American Health Organization, and WHO to carry out demographic and epidemiological studies of induced illegal abortions, and the "long term effect [population increase] could have on the social and economic development of the countries of the Western Hemisphere."

Shortly thereafter, in 1964, Peru, which in 1962 had consistently opposed the right of the United Nations to give technical assistance for population problems, established a Center for Studies on Population and Development and in 1965 sponsored a week-long conference on Peruvian population problems. Venezuela, which in 1964 reported to the United Nations that it "considered population increase, in general, as a positive factor in economic development,"[25] early in 1965 established a Department of Population in the Ministry of Public Health, early in 1966 held a large conference on population problems and public health, and in 1967 played host and cosponsor for the OAS

[24] Eighth Plenary Session of the Sixteenth Meeting of the Directing Council of the Pan American Health Organization (September-October 1965).

[25] U.N. Economic and Social Council, Inquiry among Governments on Problems Resulting from the Interaction of Economic Development and Population Changes, 64-26191 (November 1964, mimeo).

Population Conference. Jamaica, whose prime minister had for years been identified as a stalwart foe of family planning, announced in 1965 a public island-wide contraceptive program with methods ranging from rhythm to intrauterine devices. Colombia, considered by many Latin Americans as the ultimate in religious conservatism, established in 1964 a Division of Population Studies within the Association of Medical Schools. The Division has received substantial foundation grants, and has developed an ambitious program of research, training, and public education. In 1966 it received $300,000 in counterpart funds to carry out family planning education for the nation's physicians in government service.[26]

When the Christian Democrats came to power in Chile, the family planning world held its collective breath, for an ambitious contraceptive program in government hospitals had been underway for the past few years, with the tacit but unofficial consent of the government. Breath-holding gave way to sighs of relief when one of the first acts of the new minister of health in 1965 was to establish an Advisory Commission on Population and the Family within the Health Department. Chile was the site for the 1967 World Conference of the International Planned Parenthood Federation.

A new consensus is emerging in Latin America, a consensus which appeared with remarkable clarity at the Pan American Assembly conference held in Cali, Colombia, in 1965. Sponsored by the University del Valle and the Colombian Association of Medical Faculties, in collaboration with the American Assembly and the Population Council, the conference was attended by about sixty distinguished Latin Americans and twenty North Americans from the fields of medicine, the social sciences, and government. After three days of intensive, small-group discussion, the conference issued a report representing the general position of the eighty delegates. Those attending the conference

[26] Cornell International Population Program, "Latin American Coverage of Population and Family Planning" (May 1967, mimeo).

were struck with the degree of consensus on the following points, which were among the recommendations adopted in the plenary session:

(1) All nations should develop population policies as an integral part of their policies on economic development.

(2) Governments should foster responsible paternity by encouraging couples to have the number of children consistent with their own ideals.

(3) Governments should make family planning services accessible to the people who desire them, and educate the people to their availability.

These remarkable statements, along with eight others published as the final report of the conference, would have been unlikely in 1964, implausible in 1960, and unthinkable in 1955.

Of course, we must not mistake words for action. Nor must we assume that "population centers" mean low birth rates. But if birth rates are to decline more rapidly than they did in other Western nations, national governments will have to act, and the kind of consensus we have been discussing is a necessary condition for that action. We must recognize, too, that the priests, physicians, and educators present at conferences represent those more liberal on these matters than is the intelligentsia in general in Latin America. Nevertheless, even among the administrative hierarchy of the Church there is increasing tolerance of discussion and action on family planning. A good case in point comes from a provincial region in Colombia—Popayán, where a team of investigators from the Universidad de Cauca recently conducted a survey on the incidence of abortion. After an upper-class woman refused to answer the interviewer's questions "until the Pope and the Church speak on this subject," the investigator called on the Archbishop and showed him some data on abortions. "The Archbishop, in the face of the statistics, and seeing that the program was not directed against the morals of his faithful, offered his collaboration, and in order to demonstrate it sent two priests (one on behalf of the Curia, the other for the Seminary) to the Family Planning Course. . . . Subsequently any women who refused to be interviewed were given the names of the priests prepared to resolve their doubts."[27]

How different this seems from the stance taken by the Catholic Church in Puerto Rico only a few years before! There is every reason to believe that Latin America will not duplicate the bloody and shameful battle over birth control fought in Puerto Rico, in the United States, and in England. Not only the Church has changed—world conditions have changed, and most of all, the pattern of the newly emerging programs of family planning in Latin America is very different from those of Europe and the United States. The private organizations which are beginning, from Honduras to Brazil, are not headed by crusading amateurs but by educators, physicians, and government officials. They tend to be dominated by men rather than women, and, if not opulent, are probably better financed than their predecessors. They have at their disposal methods not only cheaper and more effective than ever before, but methods not connected with the sexual act itself. Demographic, medical, and social research technology is much more in evidence than was the case with earlier movements in other nations. In short, there is every reason to be optimistic not only about the organization of family planning programs, but the viability of the private organizations which support them. Given the growing receptivity of governments to the idea of population planning, it is not unlikely that the next decade will see a number of national programs supported by state funds.

Foreign Aid and Population Control

An important warning note was struck by one of the resolutions at the Cali conference: "Recognition of the dangers of population growth and formulation of the policies which may

[27] Braulio Lara Álvarez, "Prevalencia del Aborto en Popayán." Paper presented at La Ceja, Colombia (October 1965, mimeo). While the honeymoon between the Church and proponents of birth control proved to be a brief one in Colombia, the separation has been surprisingly amicable thus far.

be applied to population problems should not divert attention from the necessity for basic social and economic reform." North Americans may wonder why such a resolution, also mentioned in the introduction to the resolutions, was necessary. To understand this, one must understand both the traditional and often justifiable suspicion Latins have of North American motives, and the dominance of Marxist philosophy among many intellectuals.

Any policy promoted by the United States in Latin America is automatically open to the suspicion of intellectuals. American scholars in Latin America were the least suspect, but that privileged position of the academic fraternity has disappeared with Project Camelot. In the field of demographic problems, while scholars have been sounding the alarm for some time, for the first time in history the United States government has officially sponsored programs encouraging population control in Latin America. While the long-range effect of the new Washington policy will doubtless be salutary, the immediate effect of the sudden and not always subtle entrance of official U.S. dollars on the scene can only be expected to cause deep suspicion on the part of Latin Americans.

U.S. motives appear especially suspect when dollars for the prevention of births are linked with cutbacks in assistance for the prevention of deaths. Thus, the then Minister of Health in Peru, Dr. Aria Stella, certainly no Marxist, made what the Peruvian magazine *Caretas* termed a "sensational revelation in 1964: "The United States is willing to help in a campaign for the control of birth; but not in one to reduce the rates of death."[28] And even the Spanish and Portuguese language weekly *Vision* incurred suspicion when it ran a cover story on population. As a Mexican journalist put it: "This magazine is another instrument used by our Northern cousin to 'help' us with their notions of morals and life 'made in the U.S.A.' "[29]

In 1962 I chided the United States for its overly sensitive

[28] "La Encuesta Hall," *Caretas* (August 28, 1964).
[29] "Observatorio," *Excelsior*, Mexico (April 13, 1965).

position on population. "The United States, so insensitive to Latin feelings in most areas in the past, has maintained a sensitivity to the assumed Latin American population values and mores which should earn the envy of every applied anthropologist."[30] Only a few years later, while it is necessary to congratulate the government on its remarkable revision of policy, it might also be reminded that a pendulum can swing as far in one direction as in another. Now the danger is in too much haste, too much money, and too much "hard sell." Certainly the United States must not avoid danger areas, but there is every reason to think carefully, to employ the best brains available, to assist to the maximum the Inter-American and international agencies, and to encourage greater utilization of private agencies and foundations in assisting Latin American nations to make their own informed decisions about population planning.

As was pointed out in Chapter 1, one of the most effective ways the United States can evidence its good faith in these matters—indeed, perhaps the *only way*—is by practicing what it preaches. The recent approbation and availability of funds for domestic programs is already being appreciated in North American centers as far-flung as Puerto Rico, where the executive director of the private Family Planning Association stated recently:

The general attitude toward the birth control type program permeates the U.S. from the President on down. We are greatly benefiting from the fact that the President has been so clearly favorable toward this kind of solution to the population problem. He has let the nation and the administration know about his feelings.[31]

It is still possible for Puerto Rico to change from a national disgrace to a U.S. showcase with respect to family planning, although it is to be noted that the funds from the Anti-Poverty

30 J. Mayone Stycos, "Population Growth and the Alliance for Progress," *Eugenics Quarterly*, IX (December 1962).
31 *San Juan Star* (June 12, 1966).

Program are going to a *private* agency. The more municipal, state, and federal funds that are expended within United States borders, the more straightforward and uncomplicated can our approach be to the rest of the hemisphere.

The Communists are currently fond of pointing out that birth control should be a spontaneous result of social and economic reform. From the comfortable vantage points of the low birth rates, massive abortion programs, and sizable contraceptive programs of Communist nations, this ideological reliance on "natural" processes may seem a little strange. Yet there is something in these warnings which cannot be ignored. Birth control is not an end in itself. Neither is it a way of avoiding other problems such as unbalanced distribution of land and wealth, the needs for general education, and the exploitation of the nation's natural resources. If programs of family planning were to divert attention from these problems, the programs would not be worth the price; for low birth rates *alone* can do little for the nation and little more for the family unless accompanied by efforts to improve other aspects of the social and economic milieu. On the other hand, improvement of social and economic conditions will be immensely facilitated by slowing down the rate of population growth.

It is really not a question of whether to deal directly with population problems—it is rather a question of how this will be done, when it will be done, and who will initiate it. If governments or other groups in the public sector do not take the lead, the people will solve the problem in their own ways and in their own time. Can Latin American nations afford a *laissez-faire* policy on family planning? I cannot answer this question for them, but I hope they will face squarely not only the demographic but the social and economic consequences of leaving the solution of this complex and massive problem to a concerned but uninformed public.

Index

abortion, 10, 11, 14, 16, 29, 46, 105, 128, 135, 145, 174, 262, 285, 294-298, 300, 303, 306, 308, 312

abstinence, sexual, 135, 174-175

Africa, 12, 13, 24, 35, 53, 54, 133, 286

age of parents: at conception, 196-197, 203, 205; at marriage, 7, 14, 28, 29, 91, 127, 204, 210, 217-218, 232, 258, 268, 285, 292

Agency for International Development, 304

agrarian reform, 51

agriculture, 25, 43, 117, 270, 277, 293-294, 303

Albania, 11

Alberdi, Juan Bautista, 39

Alliance for Progress, 303, 305

altitude, effect on fertility, 226-227

Álvarez, Amezquita, Dr. José, 44-45

Amadeo, Mario, 39n, 40

American Academy of Arts and Sciences, 20

anthropology, 20, 117

anti-Americanism, 109, 310-312

Anti-Poverty Program, 115, 311-312

Antofagasta, Chile, 295

arable land, 22

Argentina, 27, 29, 33, 35, 39, 40, 42, 48, 54, 55, 62, 202n, 251, 254, 255, 269, 270, 273n, 274, 277, 278, 284n, 285, 291, 292, 297, 308; see also Buenos Aires

Arias Stella, Dr., 310

artificial insemination, 109

Asia, 24, 34, 36, 50, 53, 54, 61, 286

Association for Family Welfare, 108, 114-115

Association of Catholic Physicians, 108

audio-visual materials, 15

Australia, 50

Aymara Indians, 228, 229

Baltimore, Md., 196n

Barbados, 8

Barranquitas, P.R., 98, 113

barriadas, 238

Belaunde, Victor, 39-40, 46

Belgrade Conference, 34

Benitez, R., 61

biological limit, 7, 292

birth control: and education, 13, 14, 15, 19, 28, 63, 75-80, 80-82, 108, 142-144, 145-146, 301; and law, 5, 105, 106, 114, 301; and politics, 20, 63, 78, 98-115; technology of, 9-10, 13, 29, 291-306; see also abortion, abstinence, contraceptives, infanticide, and spacing children

Bogotá, 164, 166, 167, 168, 172, 175, 176-178, 179, 181, 256, 299, 302

Bogue, D.J., 252, 273n

Bolivia, 54-55, 254, 255, 274, 278

Brazil, 21, 34, 35, 37, 39, 55, 62, 165, 166, 250, 273n, 274, 297; see also Rio de Janeiro

breast-feeding, 8, 281

Buenos Aires, 296, 300

Cali, Colombia, Conference, 307, 309-310

Canada, 23, 35

cancer, fear of, 73-74, 79, 112

capital shortage, 20, 52

capitalism, 15-16

Caracas, Venezuela, 164, 167, 168, 172, 176, 177, 179, 180, 182, 256, 297, 298

Cardinals, College of, 169

313